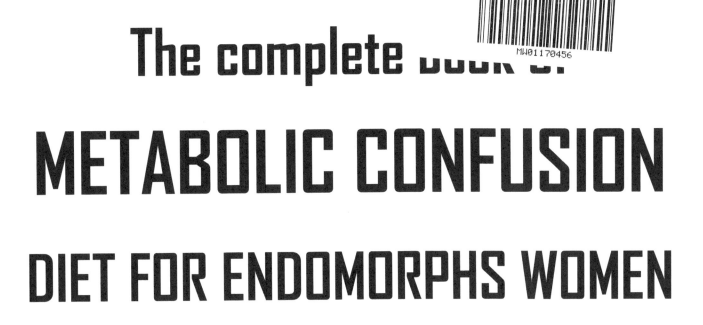

The complete BOOK OF

METABOLIC CONFUSION

DIET FOR ENDOMORPHS WOMEN

You Can Achieve a Healthier, Fitter You at Any Age with the Help of This Weight Loss Guide, Healthy Eating Meal Plan, and Delicious Cooking Methods.

Christopher Lorry

About the author

Christopher Lorry was born in San Francisco in 1985. He is a dietitian and nutritionist from the USA. He graduated in Nutrition and Food Science at the University of North Carolina. Then he worked under a health specialist for 5 years. This book is part of his passion of writing and personal experiences.

Table Of Contents

INTRODUCTION

Welcome to "The Complete Guide to a Metabolic Confusion Diet for Endomorphic Women." We've designed this book to equip you with the knowledge and tools you need to transform your body and health using the innovative metabolic confusion approach. Understanding your unique body type is crucial to achieving optimal wellness, and for endomorphs, this journey requires a tailored strategy.

Endomorphic women often face unique challenges when it comes to weight management and metabolic health. Characterized by a higher propensity to store fat, a naturally slower metabolism, and a tendency towards carbohydrate sensitivity, endomorphs can find traditional diets less effective. This book aims to address these challenges head-on with a scientifically-backed, practical approach to dieting that keeps your metabolism engaged and your body constantly adapting.

Known as calorie cycling or carb cycling, the concept of metabolic confusion is a dynamic method that aims to prevent metabolic slowdown and promote continuous fat loss. By varying your caloric and macronutrient intake throughout the week, you can keep your metabolism guessing and prevent the plateaus commonly associated with conventional dieting. This is a great method for endomorphic women since it improves metabolic health in addition to helping with weight reduction.

In the pages that follow, you will find a comprehensive guide that covers all aspects of the metabolic confusion diet. Every chapter is designed to help you on your path to becoming a better, more energetic version of yourself. From comprehending the science behind it all too provides doable food plans, Cooking Method's, and workout regimens. We'll delve into the specifics of nutrient timing, the importance of exercise, and lifestyle modifications that can further enhance your results.

Our goal is to provide you with a sustainable, flexible diet plan that adapts to your needs and lifestyle. One may attain enduring change with commitment and appropriate direction. Let's go on this adventure together and discover how your metabolism can reach its maximum potential.

PART 1: Metabolic Confusion Diet Fundamentals

Concepts and benefits

Calorie cycling, also known as carb cycling or metabolic confusion, is an innovative dietary approach that aims to prevent the body from adapting to a consistent caloric intake. Traditional diets often involve a steady reduction in calories, which can lead to a decrease in metabolic rate as the body adapts to conserve energy. Metabolic confusion disrupts this adaptation by varying daily or weekly caloric and macronutrient intake, thereby keeping the metabolism active and engaged.

The primary benefit of this approach is the prevention of metabolic slowdown, which is a common pitfall in many weight loss efforts. The body stays in a state of ambiguity when high-calorie and low-calorie, or high-carb and low-carb, **Day** s are alternated, which encourages constant fat burning and energy expenditure. This method also allows for greater dietary flexibility and sustainability, as it incorporates a variety of foods and avoids prolonged deprivation.

Comparison with Other Diets

Metabolic confusion stands apart from traditional diets such as keto, low-carb, and intermittent fasting.

- **Keto Diet:** The goal of the ketogenic diet is to put the body into a state of ketosis—where it burns fat for energy—by consuming a lot of fat and few carbs. It may be restricting and difficult to maintain over time, even though it works for some people. On the other hand, metabolic confusion allows for occasional high-carb **Day** s, which increases dietary flexibility and lowers the risk of nutritional shortages.

- **Low-Carb Diet**: Carbohydrate consumption is restricted on low-carb diets in order to lower insulin levels and encourage fat loss. However, they can lead to a decrease in metabolic rate over time. Metabolic confusion is mitigated by cycling carbohydrate intake, which prevents the body from becoming overly efficient at conserving energy.

- **Intermittent Fasting**: Times of fasting are interspersed with times of eating on this regimen. While it may be effective for some, it may not suit everyone's lifestyle or hunger patterns. Metabolic confusion, on the other hand, provides regular meals with varying macronutrient compositions, making it more adaptable to individual preferences and schedules.

Scientific Basis

Numerous research studies and scientific findings validate the principles of metabolic confusion. One significant aspect is the impact of calorie cycling on metabolism and fat loss. Studies have shown that intermittent caloric restriction can help maintain a higher metabolic rate compared to continuous calorie restriction. This strategy promotes fat loss while maintaining muscle mass because it keeps the body from going into a protracted state of caloric deficit, which often causes muscle breakdown and a slowed metabolism.

Research also highlights the hormonal benefits of metabolic confusion. Alternating between different levels of caloric and carbohydrate intake can positively influence hormones such as leptin, ghrelin, and insulin.

Leptin is regulate hunger and energy balance, tends to decrease with prolonged calorie restriction, leading to increased hunger and a lower metabolic rate. By incorporating high-calorie **Day** s, we can maintain leptin levels and support long-term weight loss and metabolic health. Moreover, cycling carbohydrate intake helps manage insulin sensitivity. On high-carb **Day** s, insulin levels rise to manage the influx of glucose, promoting glycogen storage and muscle recovery. On low-carb **Day** s, reduced insulin levels encourage fat oxidation and energy expenditure. This balance helps in optimizing both muscle gain and fat loss.

In summary, the metabolic confusion diet leverages the body's adaptive mechanisms to prevent metabolic slowdown and promote continuous fat loss. By varying caloric and macronutrient intake, it keeps the metabolism active and responsive. This is a useful and long-lasting dietary plan for endomorphic women since it promotes overall metabolic health in addition to helping with weight reduction.

Macronutrient Balance

Achieving the proper ratio of proteins, lipids, and carbs is crucial for endomorphic women in order to effectively control their weight and maintain good general health. Understanding the unique roles that each macronutrient performs in the body can help you design a diet that will support your metabolic objectives.

Proteins: For the maintenance, development, and repair of muscles, proteins are essential. They provide a feeling of satiety, helping to control appetite and reduce overall caloric intake. For endomorphs, a higher protein intake can support lean muscle mass, which in turn boosts metabolic rate. Lean meats, chicken, fish, eggs, dairy products, legumes, and plant-based proteins like quinoa and tofu are good sources of high-quality protein.

Fats: The synthesis of hormones, mental health, and the absorption of fat-soluble vitamins all depend on fats. Healthy fats from foods like avocados, nuts, seeds, olive oil, and fatty seafood should be a part of the diet. These fats have the ability to reduce inflammation and provide you with sustained energy. Prioritizing unsaturated fats over Tran's fats and too much saturated fat is crucial.

Carbohydrates: The body uses carbohydrates as its main energy source, especially while engaging in high-intensity activities. Selecting the correct kind of carbs is essential for endomorphs. Complex carbohydrates, which are high in fiber and nutrients, should be preferred by endomorphs over simple, refined carbohydrates. Vegetables, fruits, whole grains, and legumes are great sources of complex carbohydrates, which lower blood sugar and provide you long-lasting energy.

Glycemic Index and Load

Managing insulin levels is particularly important for endomorphs, who are often more sensitive to carbohydrates. The glycemic load (GL) takes into account a meal's amount and quality of carbohydrates, while the glycemic index (GI) gauges how rapidly a food elevates blood sugar levels.

Foods GI: Foods with a GI of 55 or below take longer to digest and absorb, which causes blood sugar and insulin levels to rise gradually. Non-starchy vegetables, the majority of fruits, legumes, and whole grains are a few examples. Including low-GI items in your diet helps to ensure prolonged energy levels, lower cravings, and keep blood sugar levels consistent.

High-GI foods: High-GI foods (70 or more) cause rapid spikes in blood sugar and insulin. These include sugary snacks, white bread, and certain processed foods. High-GI foods can lead to quick energy crashes and increased fat storage, making them less suitable for endomorphs that need to manage insulin sensitivity.

Glycemic load: Glycemic load (GL) provides a more accurate picture by taking into account the portion size of a carbohydrate-containing food. It is computed by taking the food's GI and multiplying it by the grams of carbs per serving, then dividing the result by 100. Ten or less is regarded as low, eleven to nineteen as medium, and twenty or more as high.

By choosing foods with a low glycemic load, endomorphs can better manage their insulin levels, reduce fat storage, and maintain steady energy throughout the day. Incorporating a variety of nutrient-dense, low-GI foods into your diet will support overall health and optimize metabolic function.

In summary, understanding macronutrient balance, calculating your caloric needs, and selecting foods based on their glycemic index and load are crucial steps for endomorphs aiming to achieve and maintain a healthy weight. By following these guidelines, you can create a sustainable nutrition plan that supports your metabolic goals and promotes long-term health.

Monitoring Progress and Staying Motivated

Starting a metabolic confusion diet involves commitment, perseverance, and a positive outlook. Sustaining motivation and tracking your progress are essential for long-term success. Here are some tips to keep you on course and recognize your accomplishments.

Tracking Your Journey

Regularly tracking your progress helps you understand how your body is responding to the diet and identify areas for improvement. Here are some effective methods:

- **Weight and Measurements**: Weekly weigh-ins and monthly measurements of your waist, hips, and other key areas can provide tangible evidence of your progress. Remember, weight can fluctuate due to a variety of factors, so focus on overall trends rather than daily changes.

- **Food Diary:** Using a nutrition app or keeping a food diary can help you monitor your caloric intake, macronutrient balance, and food choices. This practice can also highlight patterns or habits that may need adjustment.

- **Photos:** Regularly taking progress photos can visually document your transformation. Sometimes changes are more noticeable in pictures than on the scale.

- **Fitness Levels**: Tracking your strength, endurance, and flexibility improvements can provide motivation and a sense of accomplishment. Record your workout routines, including weights lifted repetitions, and any new fitness milestones.

Adjusting the Plan

Your body's requirements may fluctuate over time; therefore, it is crucial to modify your diet and exercise regimen as necessary.

- **Plateaus**: If you hit a weight loss plateau, consider changing your caloric intake, macronutrient ratios, or exercise routine. Small adjustments can reignite your progress.

- **Feedback:** Take note of your body's cues and make the necessary adjustments. Review your strategy and make the required adjustments if you're feeling worn out or aren't getting the results you want. Seeking advice from a dietician or fitness expert might provide tailored direction.

- **Goals**: Your objectives may change as you go. Whether your goal is to maintain your current weight, gain muscle, or increase your endurance, modify your strategy to suit your new goals.

Staying Motivated

Maintaining motivation is a key to long-term success. Here are some tips to keep you inspired:

- **Set realistic goals:** Establish short-term and long-term goals that are specific, measurable, and achievable. Celebrate small victories along the way to stay encouraged.

- **Find a Support System**: Surround yourself with supportive friends, family, or online communities. One way to stay accountable and find encouragement is to share your journey with others.

- **Reward Yourself**: Plan non-food rewards for reaching milestones, such as a new workout outfit, a relaxing massage, or a fun activity. Rewards can reinforce positive behavior and provide something to look forward to.

- **Stay positive**: Pay more attention to the progress you're making than to any obstacles. Remind yourself to be patient with yourself and that change takes time.

- **Variety and Fun:** Ensure that your meals and workouts are varied and enjoyable. Experiment with new Cooking Method's, try different forms of exercise, and keeps your routine engaging to avoid boredom.

- **Reflect and Reassess**: Regularly reflect on your journey and reassess your goals and strategies. Staying connected to your purpose and acknowledging your achievements can keep your motivation high.

By consistently monitoring your progress and maintaining a positive, flexible approach, you can stay motivated and achieve lasting success on the metabolic confusion diet. Embrace the journey with patience and persistence, and celebrate every step towards a healthier, more vibrant you.

PART 2: THE COOKING METHODS

BREAKFAST

1. Baked Egg Cups

What we need:

- Onion (1/3 cup)
- 12 eggs
- Bell pepper
- Bacon (6 slices)
- Mushrooms (1/3 cup)
- Black pepper (¼ tsp)

Cooking Method:

1. Begin with the burner or oven. Grease and line a 12-cup muffin pan. Try greasing the paper liners.

2. Cook chopped onions in a cooker for 15 minutes until transparent and golden. Keep aside. Thoroughly whisk the eggs. Ground black pepper flavors.

3. Make crisp bacon in a separate pan over low heat. Remove bacon from skillet and cool. Room-temperature bacon chops.

4. Combine eggs, crumbled bacon, mushrooms, bell peppers, and onions. Mix well. Fill each muffin cup 75% with the egg mixture.

5. Roast the muffin pan for 20-25 minutes in the preheated oven until the egg cups are firm and the tops are gently browned.

6. Cool the cooked egg cups for a few minutes after removing them from the oven. Place the fried egg cups on the serving tray after carefully removing them from the muffin pan.

7. Serve warm, baked egg cups for a protein-rich breakfast or brunch.

8. Serve egg cups with bread, salad leaves, or your preferred spicy sauce.

2. Browned Butter Mocha Latte

What we need:

- Unsalted butter (2 tbsp.)
- 1 ¼ cups unsweetened cashew milk
- 2 tbsp. of unsweetened cocoa powder
- 2 tbsp. sugar
- 3 tbsp. of hot fermented decaf coffee
- Special equipment (discretionary)
- Immersion blender

Cooking Method:

1. Heat butter in a saucepan over high heat until foaming and black specks emerges, indicating browning. It should take five minutes. Heat butter-seasoned coconut oil till soft.
2. Lower the heat to medium and slowly pour the cashew milk into the browned butter, stirring until it sizzles.
3. Stir in the cocoa powder and sugar. Whenever desired, use an infusion blender and mix until the blend takes the shape of a foamy latte, approximately 1 minute.
4. Empty the coffee into a giant cup. Add the hot milk mixture and mix well. Serve promptly, garnished with whipped cream and a sprinkle of unsweetened cocoa powder, if desired.

3. Sausage and Egg Sandwich

What we need:

- Cooking spray
- Turkey sausage (One patty)
- Liquid egg substitute (¼ cup)
- Bread
- Cheddar cheese (1 tbsp)

Cooking Method:

1. Spray a small, non-stick pan before preheating it in the oven. Brown all sides and cook the turkey sausage patty according to the package instructions.
2. While the sausage cooks, whisk the egg replacement in a small bowl until incorporated.

3. Put the cooked sausage on a dish and wait. Spray the skillet with extra cooking spray and add the liquid egg replacement.

4. Using a spatula, carefully whisk the egg replacement until scrambled and cooked. In the meantime, toast or broil the bread to your preference. You may need to toast the bread for a few minutes or a few minutes and a half.

5. Place the cooked turkey sausage patty on one side of the toasted bread. Place a dollop of scrambled egg substitute on the sausage patty.

6. Sprinkle cheddar cheese atop scrambled eggs. The second slice of bread covers the sandwich.

7. Right away, the sausage and egg sandwich is a nice breakfast or brunch option.

4. Fermented Carrots

What we need:

- 1 clove garlic, diced
- 1 tbsp. of sea salt
- 4–5 medium-sized carrots, skinned and grated
- 1 tbsp. freshly chopped ginger

Cooking Method:

1. Mix grated garlic, sea salt, ginger, and carrots into a big bowl.

2. Mix nicely until the salt is evenly disseminated and the carrots are barely muffled.

3. Move the combination to a pot.

4. Using a wooden scoop or your hand, depress down on the combination to remove any mood pockets, and press the brine to increase beyond the deck of the vegetables.

5. Secure the cover tightly and let it sit at room temperature for 1-2 **Day** s, or until the fermentation reaches the desired level.

6. Store in the fridge for up to 2 months.

5. Fermented Cabbage

What we need:

- 1 tbsp. of sea salt
- 1 head of cabbage, thinly diced

Cooking Method:

1. In a big bowl, mix chopped cabbage with sea salt.

2. Rub the mixture with your fingers for ten to fifteen minutes or until the brine begins to develop and the cabbage starts to fade.

3. Move the combination to a jar.

4. Gently press down on the mixture to eliminate any airbags and encourage the briny to rise beyond the vegetables' level.

5. Fasten the cover tightly and leave it at room temperature for 2–5 Day s or until the selected level of fermentation is achieved.

6. Store in the fridge for up to 2 months.

6. High-cruciferous juice

What we need:

- Three medium carrots
- Broccoli (2 cups)
- One apple, cored.
- Three cauliflower florets
- Watercress with stems (⅔ cup)

Cooking Method:

1. Scrub every fruit and vegetable under cold water. To fit in your juicer, you must peel and chop the carrots.

2. Split broccoli florets to make them easier to handle. Cut the apple into wedges after coring. Split cauliflower florets.

3. Remember to include the stems when calculating watercress amounts because they contain nutrients.

4. Build your juicer according to the manufacturer's instructions. Start by juicing carrots, broccoli, apples, cauliflower, and watercress individually. Continue until all ingredients are utilized.

5. Swirl the juice in a pitcher or jar to mix the flavors. After juicing everything, filter the high-cruciferous juice into a glass and serve.

6. To distribute nutrients equally, stir it briefly before serving. Consume high-cruciferous juice immediately to maximize its bright flavors and nutrients.

7. Fermented Beetroot

What we need:

- 1 tsp. of caraway seeds
- 1 tbsp. salt
- 3 small-sized beetroots, skinned and grated

Cooking Method:

1. Mix grated beetroots, sea salt, and caraway seeds in a big bowl.
2. Mix well until the sea salt dissolves and the beetroots begin to soften slightly.
3. Move the combination to a pot.
4. Using your fingers, push down the combination to remove any airbags, and press the briny to increase beyond the deck of the vegetables.

8.   Fermented green beans

What we need:

- 3 minced garlic cloves
- ½ tbsp. salt
- 2 cups fried beans, cut into pieces

Cooking Method:

1. Combine green beans, sea salt, and chopped garlic in a big bowl.
2. Combine nicely until the salt is evenly spread and the beans are barely muffled.
3. Move the combination to a jar.
4. Using your fingers, gently press down on the mixture to eliminate any airbags and encourage the briny to expand beyond the vegetables.

9.Fermented Zucchini

What we need:

- 1 tsp. dried oregano
- 1 tbsp. of paper and sea salt
- 3 small-sized zucchinis, slashed into rounds

Cooking Method:

1. Mix slashed zucchini, sea salt, and dried oregano.
2. Combine well until the salt is evenly dispersed and the zucchini is barely cushioned.
3. Move the combination into a jar.
4. Utilizing an unbending scoop, push down on the combination to remove any airbags and press the briny to increase beyond the deck of the vegetables.
5. Fasten the cover tightly and keep it until the desired level of fermentation is reached.
6. Stock in the fridge for up to 2 months.

10.   Pineapple and blueberry smoothie

What we need:

- Pineapple chunks (½ cup)
- ½ apples
- Frozen blueberries (1 cup)
- English cucumber (½ cup)
- ½ cup of water

Cooking Method:

1. Blend pineapple pieces, sliced apple, frozen blueberries, chopped English cucumber, and water. Blend smooth.
2. Blend all ingredients at high speed until creamy. If necessary, take a break and scrape the blender to mix all the contents.
3. Continue mixing until the mixture is silky. Try some smoothies and add fruit or water if you prefer them sweeter or thicker.
4. Pour the pineapple and blueberry smoothie into a glass after adjusting the consistency. Add a pineapple slice or blueberries to enhance the dish's presentation.

5. Serve the smoothie right away so your visitors can enjoy the pineapple, blueberries, apple, and cucumber flavors. Taste the smoothie's luscious flavor and blueberries' antioxidant properties with every drink.

11.   Corn Pudding

What we need:

- Unsalted butter (3 tbsp.)
- 3 eggs
- Granulated sugar (2 tbsp.)
- Baking soda substitute (½ tsp.)
- 2 tbsp. of flour
- Frozen corn kernels (2 cups)
- Rice milk (¾ cup)
- Light sour cream (2 tbsp.)

Cooking Method:

1. Butter or spray a baking dish or ramekins, and preheat the oven. A microwave-safe bowl melts unsalted butter best. Even the stove is useful.

2. In another bowl, beat eggs and sugar until the sugar lines disappear. Mix eggs and melted butter until lump-free.

3. Stir baking soda and flour into the batter. Smoothen one cup of frozen corn kernels in a mixer. In a separate dish, beat the eggs before adding the corn mush and remaining

4. Combine the kernels, rice milk, and light sour cream. Make sure everything mixes. Pour or divide the batter into ramekins or baking dishes.

5. For the ideal texture and brown topping, move the pudding to ramekins or a baking dish and boil for 45 minutes. Before consuming, take the corn pudding out of the oven and allow it to cool.

6. Corn pudding can be reheated for dessert or as a as a side dish. Before serving, sprinkle powdered sugar or whipped cream to make the meal look luxurious.

7. Delicious, creamy corn pudding.

12. Egg and avocado salad

What we need:

- 1 avocado, mashed
- 2 boiled eggs, diced
- pepper and to taste
- salt
- 1 tbsp. of lime sap
- Fresh cilantro

Cooking Method:

1. Combine the diced boiled eggs with smashed avocado in a big bowl.
2. Add lime juice, diced cilantro, pepper, and salt.
3. Combine everything until well-mixed.
4. Serve on a lettuce-covered mattress or with your favorite GAPS-friendly hacks.

13. Eggs and vegetables

- **What we need:**
- 1/4 cup minced onion
- Salt and pepper
- 2 cups chopped cucumber
- 2 tbsp. of lemon sap
- 1 cup sliced red bell pepper
- 2 boiled eggs, sliced
- Coconut oil 2 tbsp.
- 1 tbsp. diced fresh parsley

Cooking Method:

1. Mix the cooked eggs with chopped cucumber, onion, and bell pepper in a dish.
2. Combine the chopped parsley, pepper, lemon juice, olive oil, and salt.
3. Combine everything until well mixed.
4. Serve on a bed of lettuce, or with your favorite GAPS-friendly pirates.

14. Omelet

What we need:

- Separate 1 tbsp. and add 1 tsp. of ghee or unsalted margarine.
- 1/4 cup diced onions
- 14 cups of cut mushrooms
- Add 2 tbsp. of diced green or red bell peppers to the
- 1/4 cup ground pork or hamburger
- 1/4 tsp. acceptable ocean salt, partitioned
- 4 enormous eggs, beaten
- 1/4 cup diced Canadian bacon
- ¼ cup destroyed sharp cheddar, in addition to extra for topping sliced green onions, for trimming
- 14 cups of salsa, for serving
- 1 cup acrid cream, for serving

Cooking Method:

1. First, in a pan over medium-low heat, melt 1 tbsp. of ghee. Toss in some ringer peppers, mushrooms, and onions and cook until they're soft.
2. Sauté ground pork for 3 minutes until done. Sprinkle 1/8 tsp. Salt.
3. Whisk together the eggs, Canadian bacon, water, and salt in a bowl until well combined.
4. Store it securely. Heat a 12-inch saucepan on medium-low heat. Swirl in the remaining of ghee.
5. Pour the egg into the blender. Spread the eggs and cook until almost set. After removing the top, sprinkle cheddar over the omelet. Spread veggie filling on cheddar.
6. Place the omelet on a serving plate with a greased center.
7. Be generous with cheddar and green onions. Serve the entrée with salsa and acrid cream.

15. The Exquisite Greek Yogurt Parfait

What we need:

- smoothly and creamy 1 cup Greek yogurt
- Add 2 tbsp. of light and pleasing honey.
- Mixed berries 1 cup
- ¼ cup of granola
- 2 tbsp. of unsweetened coconut flakes, toasted
- 2 tbsp. of chopped nuts
- Mint leaves are fresh.

Cooking Method:

1. Mix Greek yogurt and honey in a bowl. Gentle stir till thoroughly combined.
1. Select a glass or parfait dish. Spoon a layer of honey-infused yogurt onto the bottom.
2. Sprinkle some fresh mixed berries on top of the yoghurt layer.
3. Cover the berries with granola.
4. Scatter toasted coconut flakes over the granola layer.
5. Layer yogurt, berries, granola, and coconut flakes until the glass is full.
6. Add a layer of chopped nuts on top for extra crunch.
7. Garnish with fresh mint leaves.
8. Serve immediately and enjoy the combination of creamy yogurt, sweet honey, fresh berries, crunchy granola, coconut flakes, and nuts.

16. Chicken Cashew

What we need:

- 1 bunch of scallions
- 2 cups of boneless, skinless, weakling thighs
- 2 tbsp. well-diced, skinned, and refreshed ginger
- Black pepper
- 1 yellow bell pepper and 1 minced celery branch
- 2 tsp. of arrowroot flour
- 3 cups of basic chicken stock

- 3 tbsp. of coconut oil
- 1 tsp. salt
- 1 cup salted, grated cashews
- 4 garlic cloves, nicely minced

Cooking Method:

1. Chop scallions, as well as different leafy and white pieces.
2. Pat weaklings parched, lacerate into a 2-inch piece, and decorate with pepper and salt.
3. Warm a skillet over a high flame.
4. Flow oil, stir, and fry the chicken until boiled for 5 minutes. Move to a receptacle.
5. Combine celery, garlic, ginger, red pepper chips, bell pepper, and scallion whites in a skillet and stir for 7 minutes until the peppers are tender.
6. Combine the soup with arrowroot flour and sauce, and then place the vegetables in a bowl.
7. Decrease warmth and simmer, sometimes provoking, until reduced.
8. Swirl in chicken, scallion greens, cashews, and any juices.

17. Quinoa Breakfast Bowl

What we need:

- ½ cup quinoa, rinsed
- 1 cup of water
- 1 cup Greek yogurt
- 1 tbsp. of honey
- ½ tsp. vanilla extract
- 1 cup mixed berries (blueberries, raspberries, strawberries)
- 2 tbsp. chopped mixed nuts (almonds, pecans, and walnuts)
- 2 tbsp. toasted, unsweetened coconut flakes
- fresh Mint leaves

Cooking Method:

1. Rinse quinoa under cold water and drain well.
1. In a pot, combine quinoa and water. Bring to a boil, and then simmer for 10 minutes until water is absorbed and the quinoa is tender. Fluff with a fork and set aside.

2. In a bowl, combine Greek yogurt, honey, and vanilla extract. Stir until smooth.

3. Spoon cooked quinoa into a serving bowl.

4. On top of the quinoa, add the yogurt mixture.

5. Add mixed berries over the yogurt and quinoa.

6. Sprinkle chopped nuts over the bowl.

7. Scatter toasted coconut flakes on top.

8. Garnish with fresh mint leaves.

9. Serve immediately and enjoy the combination of quinoa, yogurt, berries, nuts, and coconut.

18. Herb Crust with Grilled Salmon

What we need:

- 4 salmon fillets
- Olive oil
- Oregano ½ cup
- One clove of garlic
- Cilantro 1/3 cup
- Green onion, ¼ cup
- Lemon juice
- Black pepper and salt

Cooking Method:

1. Prepare an individual pouch out of the aluminum foil for each fillet, and have them on hand.

2. Utilizing a blender, thoroughly incorporate the oregano, salt, onion, pepper, cilantro, garlic, lemon juice, and olive oil until everything is uniform in texture and flavor. Mix well until there are no longer any lumps.

3. After completing those steps, re-stitch the pocket and evenly distribute the contents throughout the fish.

4. Cook for about 35 minutes at 350 degrees in a preheated oven.

19.   Carb Gumbo with Seafood

What we need:

- Twenty ounces of okra
- One pound of skinless and boneless chicken thighs has been cut into pieces
- 10-ounces of shrimp after being cooked
- A chicken broth is equivalent to two cups.
- Measure out a half tsp. of cayenne pepper.
- 2 cups of tomato sauce with no added sugar
- 2 celery stalks, diced, are included.
- 1 ½ cups of thinly sliced onions
- 2 diced sausages
- 2 bay leaves in the bud
- Cut and seed one cup of green bell peppers.
- Use pepper and salt as needed.
- Smash three cloves of garlic.
- 1 tsp. of dried onion flakes.

Cooking Method:

1. All ingredients except shrimp should be mixed in the cooker.
2. The pan's lid should be in close proximity.
3. The process involves cooking at a low temperature for six to eight hours.
4. Then, swirl it into your precooked shrimp ten minutes before the end of the time allotment.
5. When serving the dish, shake some Seatrain's over it.
6. 6. Serve with cauliflower-based rice.

20.   Egg and Avocado Salad

What we need:

- 1 avocado, smashed
- 2 boiled eggs, diced
- Pepper and salt as your taste
- 2 tbsp. lime juice
- Fresh cilantro

Cooking Method:

1. Combine the diced boiled eggs with smashed avocado in a big bowl.
2. Add lime juice, diced cilantro, pepper, and salt.
3. Combine everything until well-mixed.
4. Serve.

21.   Egg and Vegetable

What we need:

- 1 tbsp. of oil
- Salt and pepper
- 2 boiled eggs, sliced
- 1 tbsp. of lemon sap
- 2 cups diced vegetables
- ¼ cup diced onion
- 1 tbsp. minced fresh parsley

Cooking Method:

1. Mix the cooked eggs with the vegetables.
2. Mix the chopped parsley, pepper, lemon juice, oil, and salt.
3. Combine everything until well mixed.
4. Serve.

22.   Meatloaf

What we need:

- One pound of ground pork
- One tsp. of paprika
- Two eggs
- 2 cups chopped onion
- 12 cups of almond flour
- One tbsp. of coconut oil
- One tbsp. of garlic powder
- One pound of ground turkey
- Six tsp. of Italian seasoning
- Two tsp. of red pepper flakes
- Use salt and pepper.

Cooking Method:

1. Pour oil into a pan and heat it up to a low-medium temperature.
2. When warm, mix the onion and heat it up until it is transparent.
3. Take it away from the heat. Add almond flour, eggs, and seasonings to a dish and stir.
4. Add meat and onions, and then combine with clean hands.
5. Shape into a loaf. Grease the cooker with coconut oil.
6. Put the loaf in your slow cooker, making sure there's at least a half-inch space between the meat and the sides of the cooker, and that the top of the loaf is flat.
7. It is situated adjacent to the cover of the pan.
8. Heat on high for 180 minutes, so that the meat reaches 150 degrees.
9. If you want the loaf to be substantial and not crumbly, let it sit in the cooker for 15–30 minutes after cooking, with the cooker turned off and the lid removed.
10. Eat!

23. Turkey Casserole

What we need:

- Ten fresh eggs
- 12-ounce turkey sausage
- One mug of no-sugar-added salsa
- One mug of heavy cream
- Salt and pepper
- One mug of Mexican cheese blended
- One tsp. of chili flexes
- Half tsp. of garlic paste
- 12 tsp. cumin

Cooking Method:

1. Heat a skillet and cook the sausage.
2. When it isn't pink, blend in salsa and seasonings.
3. Put out from warmth.
4. Take a dish and beat the eggs and milk as needed.
5. Mix the pork as well as the cheese, and stir.
6. Prepare a crockpot with a coconut-oil-based cooking spray.
7. Pour in the casserole and close the cover.
8. Heat on low for five hours, or if you want to eat sooner, on high for 2–12 hours.

24. Almond-Cranberry Cereal Bar

What we need:

- Almond margarine (½ cup)
- Sugar (2/3 cup)
- 5 cups of fresh wheat grain squares
- Dried cranberries (3/4 cup)
- ½ cup fragmented almonds, toasted
- Cooking shower

Cooking Method:

1. Spoon almond margarine and honey into a large Dutch broiler. Boil on medium heat. Blend with oats, cranberries, and almonds, hurling to coat.

2. Put the blend into a prepared dish covered with a cooking splash, squeezing it into an even layer with cling wrap.

3. Let stand 1 hour so that sets. Cut it into 12 bars.

25. Mediterranean Chickpea Flour Frittata

Cooking Method:

- 1 cup chickpea flour
- 2 tbsp. yeast
- 1 bell pepper, sliced
- pepper
- 1 ¼ cups water
- Powdered turmeric ½ tsp.
- baking powder
- diced 1 onion
- 2 tbsp. oil
- chopped green coriander
- 1 zucchini, diced
- ¼ cup sliced black olives

Cooking Method:

1. Pour flour, salt, pepper, yeast, baking powder, water, and turmeric into a large dish and mix until smooth. Reserve for set.
2. Warm butter in a cooker. Stir chopped onion and pepper so that soften. Swirl diced zucchini for some minutes until tender.
3. Simmer cherry tomatoes and black olives for 2 minutes. Spread chickpea flour batter evenly over cooker-roasted veggies.
4. Bake the cooker frittata until firm and golden brown in the Warmed oven.
5. The frittata should cool after removing the pan from the oven. Add fresh, chopped parsley before serving.
6. Slice the Mediterranean Chickpea Flour Frittata with Roasted Veggies and serve warm.

26.   Cappuccino Chocolate Chip Muffin

What we need:

- Cooking shower
- 1 and 3/4 cups low-fat heating blend
- Sugar (½ cup)
- ½ cup of high-temperature water
- 2 tbsp. of instant coffee granules
- Canola oil (1/4 cup)
- One enormous egg
- Half a cup of semisweet chocolate is smaller than regular chips.

Cooking Method:

1. Preheat the broiler to 400°.
2. Put ½ paper biscuit cup liners in the biscuit cups; coat them with cooking spray.
3. Put the mixture into dry measuring cups, being careful to keep the cups level with the blade. Whisk the heating mixture and sugar together in a medium bowl.
4. Join ½ cups of high-temperature water and espresso granules, blending until the espresso breaks down. Consolidate the oil and egg, mixing with a whisk; mix in an espresso blend. Add the espresso blend to the heating blend, mixing just until sodden. Blend in chocolate-scaled-down chips.
5. Gently spoon the player into the arranged liners. Heat it for 20 minutes at 400°F or until the biscuits spring back when contacted softly. Expel the biscuits from the container quickly and put them on a line rack. Serve warm.

27.   Berry Crumble Pudding

What we need:

Filling:

- Almond milk 1 cup
- 2 cups of water
- ¼ mugs of chia seeds
- of mixed berries 1 cup
- 1 tsp. of cinnamon
- ½ tsp. of pure vanilla essence

- A dash of sea salt

Topping:

- ½ cups almond flour (blanched)
- 1 cup plain whole-fat yogurt
- ¼ cups unsweetened shredded coconut
- 1 cup granulated stevia
- 1 tsp. of cinnamon
- 1 tsp. of pure vanilla essence

Cooking Method:

1. Mix water, milk, chia seeds, psyllium husk, cinnamon, salt, and vanilla essence in your slow cooker.
2. Add berries on top, but do not mix.
3. In a dish, combine the coating components.
4. Spread it on the upper part of the crumble and adjacent to the cover of the pan.
5. Bring it to a simmer and cook for four hours, covered.
6. When time is up, turn off the cooker (keep the lid on) and wait an hour before serving!

28.   Chewy Date-Apple Bars

What we need:

- Two and a half cups for the entire set of dates
- 1 cup of dried apples
- Pecans, toasted (½ cup)
- Rolled oats (½ cup)
- Ground cinnamon (1/4 tsp.)

Cooking Method:

1. Bring the oven down to 350 degrees.
2. Put the initial three ingredients into a blender and mix until the leafy foods are finely slashed.
3. Include oats and cinnamon; beat 8 to multiple times or until soggy and oats are cleaved. Blend into a delicately lubed 9 x 5-inch portion container, squeezing into an even layer with a saran cover.

4. Heat for 15 minutes at 350°F. Cool completely in a dish on a line rack. Then cut into 12 bars.

29.   Waffle Sandwich

What we need:

- 1 (1.33-ounce) solidified multigrain waffle
- 2 tbsp. cream cheese, mollified
- 2 tsp. of dark-colored sugar
- Ground cinnamon (¼ tsp.)
- 1 tbsp. of raisins
- 1 tbsp. hacked pecans, toasted

Cooking Method:

1. Toast waffles as per bundle headings.
2. Blend cream cheese, dark sugar, and cinnamon until very well mixed. Spread the cream cheese blend over the waffles. Sprinkle with raisins and pecans.
3. Cut the waffle down the middle. Place the waffle parts together, ensuring the filling is inside.

30.   Veggie Breakfast Scramble

What we need:

- For a smooth and protein-packed base, lightly batter six large eggs.
- 2 tbsp. of olive oil for a gentle glaze.
- 1 cup of spinach leaves, roughly diced, for a vibrant explosion of green
- For a sweet and savory base, finely chop one small onion.
- 1 clove of garlic, minced for some hint of aromatic appeal
- Pepper and salt, to taste, for a harmonious balance of flavors
- Diced fresh parsley serves as a final embellishment for herbal witchcraft.
- 1 chopped red bell pepper for a burst of vibrant sweetness.
- 1 yellow bell pepper, diced
- 1 zucchini, thinly cut, for a vital green element
- 1 cup of cherry tomatoes, halved, for fleshy distinction shots

Cooking Method:

1. Cooking oil glazes and enhances flavor. Sear the finely sliced onion slowly in the pan since it smells pungent.

2. Gently combining crushed garlic eliminates its beautiful fragrance and perfumes the air.

3. Add chopped red and yellow bell peppers to the pan with onions and garlic. Watch the symphony's fiery colors.

4. Carefully stir the zucchini into the skillet. Refresh the meal with its gentleness. Season veggies with pepper and salt to invigorate and modify taste.

5. For exquisite sweetness, carefully add split cherry tomatoes with their luscious saps.

6. As the veggies dance and their vibrant green colors mix, add roughly chopped spinach leaves to the pan.

7. Prepare a skillet for soft-beaten eggs. Encourage them to embrace the mixture's essence and accept the veggie costume's smooth surface.

8. Beat the eggs gently and add them to the colorful mixture. The beautiful, delicious veggies make you want fluffy eggs.

9. Stir and tuck the mixture until the eggs are cooked, the flavors are blended, and the colors are bright.

10. With fresh parsley, the scramble tastes herbaceous.

11. Transition breakfast to veggies. Master scrambled eggs in the morning.

31.   Poha

Cooking Method:

- ½ tsp. mustard seeds
- 1 cup flattened rice (Poha)
- 2 tbsp. ghee
- Powder Turmeric, and black salt to taste
- ½ tsp. cumin seeds
- Chopped mixed vegetables (e.g., peas, carrots, bell peppers)
- A few curry leaves
- Fresh basil for garnish

Cooking method:

1. The rice that has been flattened, also known as Poha, has to be rinsed in cold water, after which it should be drained and then keep aside.

2. Add the mustard and cumin to the pan when the ghee or oil has reached the desired temperature.

3. Curry leaves should be added to the vegetables while they are being sautéed and cooked until the vegetables have lost some of their crispness.

4. Combine the turmeric powder, the ordinary table salt, and the black table salt in a mixing bowl.

5. After giving the Poha a quick rinse, mix it with the other ingredients and give everything a good toss.

32.   Bagel Sandwich

What we need:

- ½ cup (4 ounces) goat cheddar, disintegrated
- 4 ounces cheese cream mollified
- 1 tbsp. of honey
- 1/3 cup hacked toasted pecans
- 1 cinnamon-raisin twirl small bagel, split and toasted
- ¼ cup red Anjou pear, unpeeled and meagerly cut

Cooking Method:

1. Consolidate the initial three ingredients in a little bowl. Mix in pecans.

2. Spread 1 tbsp. of goat cheddar uniformly onto the cut sides of the bagel.

3. Spot pear cuts on the base portion of the bagel. Supplant the bagel top.

4. Spread and chill, staying spread for as long as a week.

33.   Poached eggs with spinach

What we need:

- 1 cup of spinach
- 2 eggs
- Pepper and salt to your taste.
- 1 tbsp. of ghee or butter

Cooking Method:

1. Warm a dish of water until it's simmering.

2. Crack the eggs into the boiling water and allow them to steam for about 3–4 minutes.

3. Warm the butter in a pan, and then swirl in the spinach until it wilts.

4. Move the cooked eggs from the boiling water with a spoon and keep them on the canopy of the spinach.

5. Add salt and pepper to taste.

34. Cauliflower and Green Bean

What we need:

- 1 cauliflower
- 1 onion, nicely diced
- Green beans, clipped
- 1 cup of almond milk
- Pepper and salt

Cooking Method:

1. Take a large cooker and boil cauliflower in vegetable broth with olive oil.

2. Mix in onions and beans and boil for a short time. Move the combination into a grinder, and mix coconut milk, salt, and pepper until smooth.

3. Mix green beans, mashed cauliflower, and toppings on aluminum foil and cook for 10 to 18 minutes at 410F.

4. Enjoy.

35. Baked Oatmeal Cups

What we need:

- 1 ½ cups oats
- 1 ½ cups unsweetened milk
- ¼ cup honey
- A little of cinnamon
- salt
- 1 large apple, skinned and grated
- Vanilla essence 1 tsp.
- ¼ cup raisins

Cooking Method:

1. Take a dish, combine old-fashioned oats, cinnamon, salt, and baking powder.

2. Take another dish, combine unsweetened almond milk, honey, and vanilla.

3. Combine the wet and dry components. Evenly distribute grated apples and raisins.

4. Overfill muffin cups with oatmeal. Roast in the oven until the tops are light brown.

5. Allow the oatmeal cups chill in the muffin tray. Cool the oatmeal cups on a wire rack before serving.

6. Apple Cinnamon Baked Oatmeal Cups with Raisins are easy and yummy!

36. Cheesy Hash with Eggs, Bacon, and Cauliflower

What we need:

- ½ cauliflower heads
- Two eggs
- Two slices of bacon
- Half a tsp. of garlic powder
- 1 cup of water
- 12 cups cheddar cheese
- 12 tbsp. of minced chives
- Half a tsp. of onion powder
- Splash of heavy cream
- Salt as needed.
- Use black pepper for testing.

Cooking Method:

1. Break up the cauliflower into florets.

2. Crack eggs into a ramekin and mix with cream, a bit of pepper, and salt as needed.

3. Transfer water into your pressure cooker and insert a steamer basket.

37.   Poached Salmon

What we need:

- 2 ounces of water
- 1 tbsp. of a dry white wine
- One bay leaf
- One slender piece of everything:
- Black peppercorns with salt in the kosher style
- 5–6 sprigs of fresh herbs (include dill, tarragon, and other similar herbs)
- 2 lb. salmon skin-on or 4-6 fillets
- Components of the Garnish
- More salt
- Black pepper that has just been freshly cracked
- Olive oil
- Wedges of lemons

Cooking Method:

1. The contents of the slow cooker should include wine, water, a bay leaf, shallots, salt, peppercorns, and herbs. Prepare for twenty-five minutes on the highest setting.

2. Salt and pepper should be sprinkled on the apex of the fish. Position it in the cooker so that the skin is facing down.

3. Cover the lid and steam for 45 minutes, checking to see whether it is done. Continue if not done until opaque, potentially up to one hour.

4. If you choose the warm setting, it is appropriate for a few hours' worth of use. Oil and other garnishes should be drizzled over the dish.

5. Enjoy!

38. Cottage Cheese with Nut Medley

What we need:

- ½ cup cottage cheese

- ¼ cup mixed nuts, roughly chopped

- ½ tsp. honey

- Fresh berries

Cooking Method:

1. Ensure you have all the ingredients ready for your cottage cheese with nuts. Scoop out the desired amount of cottage cheese and put it in a dish.

2. Roughly chop the variety of nuts of your choice. Almonds, walnuts, and pecans work wonderfully together, providing a mix of textures and flavors. Sprinkle the chopped nuts over the cottage cheese.

3. If you desire a touch of sweetness, add honey over the cottage cheese and nut mixture. Adjust the amount to your taste preference, or skip it altogether if you prefer a more savory dish.

4. For an extra burst of color, flavor, and nutrition, adds a handful of fresh berries on top. Strawberries, blueberries, and raspberries complement the creaminess of the cottage cheese and the crunch of the nuts.

5. Your Cottage Cheese with Nut Medley is ready to enjoy. Each spoonful combines the creamy richness of cottage cheese with the satisfying crunch of mixed nuts and the subtle sweetness of honey (if used). The addition of fresh berries adds a delightful contrast of juiciness and tanginess.

6. Feel free to get creative with your cottage cheese and nut medley. Experiment with different nut varieties, adjust the sweetness level, or try different combinations of fresh fruits.

39. Almond Oats

Cooking Method:

- ½ cup rolled oats
- 2 tbsp. chocolate chips
- ½ cup any milk
- 1 tbsp. oil
- Honey 1 tbsp.
- crushed almonds
- Shredded coconut 1 tbsp.
- Optional toppings: additional shredded coconut, chocolate chips, sliced almonds

Cooking Method:

1. Mix oats, almond milk, almond butter, shredded coconut, chocolate chips, and sliced almonds in a jar.

2. Mix everything well. Refrigerate overnight to soften the oats.

3. Stir the overnight oats in the morning.

4. Add shredded coconut, chocolate chips, and sliced almonds to Almond Joy Overnight Oats before serving.

5. Enjoy these tasty and handy overnight oats in the fridge!

40. Tofu and Veggie Breakfast Burrito

Cooking Method:

- 1 tbsp. melted butter
- ½ cup firm tofu, diced
- 1 cup cooked quinoa
- ½ tsp. powdered cumin
- ½ cup corn kernels (fresh, canned, or fresh)
- Salt
- Fresh coriander leaves, chopped
- ¼ cup salsa verde (store-bought or homemade)
- ¼ cup diced bell peppers (any color)

- Lime wedges (for serving)
- ¼ cup minced onion

Cooking Method:

1. Warm melted butter in a cooker on medium. Season cubed tofu with cumin, paprika, pepper, and salt. Tofu should be golden brown and slightly crispy after 5-7 minutes of stirring.

2. Add black beans, corn kernels, diced bell peppers, and minced onion to the tofu cooker.

3. Continue cooking for 5 minutes to tenderize veggies. Serve bowls of cooked quinoa. Put tofu and veggies on top.

4. Pour verde salsa on bowls.

5. Serve lime wedges and chopped cilantro separately.

6. Veggie and Tofu Breakfast Burrito Bowl with Salsa Verde is a healthy breakfast

LUNCH

41.   Spicy Pumpkin

Elements:

- 3 cups of water
- 1 cup diced oats
- ¼ cup chopped pecans
- Allspice
- 1 cup pumpkin pulp
- ½ cup sugar

Cooking Method:

1. Flow the water into the cooker.

2. Mix all the elements with the water in a heat-proof dish and arrange them in the steamer stands.

3. Reduce the stands in the cooker and close the cover.

4. Cook on high pressure for 3 minutes.

5. Turn off the flame and wait for the cooker to calm down.

6. Combine the elements in a little dish.

7. At the serving time, if required, mix a bit of almond juice with the ready oatmeal.

42. Grilled Chicken and Avocado Salad

What we need:

For the salad:

- 3 skinless, boneless breasts of chicken
- 6 cups mixed leaves: spinach, arugula, or your favorite green salad
- 1 ripe, minced avocado
- ½ chopped cucumber
- 1 cup halved tomatoes
- ¼ thinly chopped onion
- Olive oil for grilling
- Salt to taste

For the salad dressing:

- Salt
- 4 tbsp. of olive oil
- 1 tbsp. balsamic vinegar
- Dijon mustard 1 tsp.
- Pepper to taste
- 1 clove of minced garlic

Cooking Method:

1. Set the temperature in your oven somewhere between high and medium. Skirmish the breasts with flavor and oil with black pepper and salt.

2. Keep the meat in the preheated oven. Bake for approximately six to seven minutes on each surface. Baking time may differ because it depends on the thickness of your chicken.

3. Let the meat cool for a few minutes after grilling to disperse dampness. Cut the grilled chicken into thin piece.

4. Put a big salad dish; combine the mixed greens, chopped avocado, cucumber, tomatoes, and onion. Take a dish and whip all the elements—mustard, olive oil, pepper, salt, vinegar, and garlic—to create the dressing in it.

5. Sprinkle the salad over the mixer and combine gently to coat the ingredients consistently. Organize the chopped chicken, which is grilled on top of the avocado salad.

6. Divide the grilled chicken and avocado salad among serving plates. Optionally, you can sprinkle some crumbled feta cheese or toasted nuts (e.g., almonds or walnuts) for added flavor and texture.

7. Serve your delicious and healthy grilled chicken and avocado salad immediately.

43. Tofu and veggie breakfast burrito

Cooking Method:

- 1 tbsp. of melted butter
- ½ cup firm tofu, diced
- 1 cup of cooked quinoa
- ½ tsp. powdered cumin
- ½ cup corn kernels (fresh, canned, or fresh)
- Salt
- Fresh coriander leaves, chopped
- ¼ cup salsa verde (store-bought or homemade)
- ¼ cup diced bell peppers (any color)
- Lime wedges (for serving)
- ¼ cup minced onion

Cooking Method:

1. Warm melted butter in a cooker on medium. Season cubed tofu with cumin, paprika, pepper, and salt. Tofu should be golden brown and slightly crispy after 5-7 minutes of stirring.

2. Add black beans, corn kernels, diced bell peppers, and minced onion to the tofu cooker.

3. Continue cooking for 5 minutes to tenderize the veggies. Serve bowls of cooked quinoa. Put tofu and veggies on top.

4. Pour the verde salsa into bowls.

5. Serve lime wedges and chopped cilantro separately.

6. A veggie and tofu burrito bowl with salsa verde is a healthy lunch.

44.   Deviled Egg with Pickled Jalapenos

What we need:

- Canola mayonnaise (¼ cup)
- Jalapeno pepper rings (2 tbsp.)
- 1 tbsp. Creole mustard
- 1 tsp. Sriracha (hot bean stew sauce)
- Ground dark pepper (¼ tsp.)
- 4 hard-cooked enormous eggs, stripped
- 4 Boston lettuce leaves
- 2 tbsp. slashed green onion tops

Cooking Method:

1. Consolidate the initial five ingredients into a bowl.

2. Cut the eggs down the middle and evacuate the yolk. Finely slash the egg white; press the yolk through a strainer using the back of a spoon.

3. Tenderly overlay the egg with the mayonnaise blend. Top every lettuce leaf with about 14 cups of mixed greens and 1 ½ tsp. of green onion tops.

45.   Adobo Chicken

What we need:

- 1 pound of chicken
- Two tbsp. of adobo sauce
- 1 tbsp. of flour
- 0.75 cups cheddar
- 0.5 cups salsa
- 1 tbsp. of butter
- 0.5 cups of milk

Cooking Method:

1. Mix adobo and salsa. Place it in the pressure cooker.

2. Add chicken. Cook on low for a total of eight hours.

3. Tear the chicken into shreds.

4. In a separate cooker, heat the butter. Mix flour.

5. Stir in milk. Stir until there are no lumps. Mix in the cheese while stirring. Continue to stir until a thick paste forms.

6. Place the mixture in the cooker.

7. Give the flavors some time to combine.

46. Beef Bread

What we need:

- Lean ground beef (1 pound)
- White vinegar
- Bread crumbs (½ cup)
- One large egg
- Chopped basil (2 tbsp.)
- ½ cup sweet onion
- 1 tsp. diced thyme
- Garlic powder
- 1 tsp. minced parsley
- ¼ tsp. of black pepper
- Brown sugar

Cooking Method:

1. After spraying or oiling a loaf cooker with butter, set it in the oven to preheat until the temperature reaches 350 degrees Fahrenheit (175 degrees Celsius).

2. Combine the ground beef, bread crumbs, egg, white vinegar, thyme, parsley, black pepper, and garlic powder in a big mixing dish.

3. Distribute the spices evenly throughout the meat by using either your clean hands or a spoon to properly combine everything.

4. Make a loaf shape with the meat combination and set it into the heated loaf pan.

5. To add a little sweetness during baking, sprinkle a thin coating of brown sugar across the meatloaf.

6. Roast the meatloaf for thirty to thirty-five minutes at the measurement temperature.

7. Wait a few minutes after taking the meatloaf out of the oven before slicing and serving.

8. Warm the delicious meatloaf pieces and serve with your preferred dishes, a healthy salad, or mashed potatoes.

9. Indulge in the savory taste of this meatloaf made with lean ground beef, fragrant herbs, and a brown sugar topping.

47. Almond with Coconut

What we need:

- ¼ cup sliced almonds and coconut flakes
- 1 cup of almond milk
- Sugar to test
- 2 cups of coconut milk

Cooking Method:

1. Flow the pints of milk into the cooker and cook.
2. Churn till it burns.
3. Count the stew and rice before closing the cover.
4. Boil for 4 minutes on medium heat.
5. Turn off the flame and wait 12 minutes.
6. Mix the vanilla and sugar.
7. Separate the lead and oats from the crushed coconut and almonds.

48. Vegan Curd

What we need:

- 1 packet of vegan curd
- 2 cups of soy milk

Cooking Method:

1. Add milk and curd.
2. Flow into a cooker you understand works in your oven. Depart off any surfaces.
3. Set it into the oven. You do not require measuring any water in the jar because it achieves an even increase in heat.
4. Go around your work until the alert rings; next, take the curd from the oven.
5. Set the cover on the receptacles, and then stock them in the cooler for at least 5 hours.

6. The curd will be very spicy, which is why it is improved with sugar, jam, fruit, and vanilla.

49. Banana Porridge

What we need:

- A dash of cinnamon
- 2 ½ cups almond juice
- 2 sliced bananas

Cooking Method:

1. Combine the bananas and milk in your cooker.
2. Close the cover.
3. Stir on a high flame for about 5 minutes.
4. Turn off the flame and permit the cooker to calm down.
5. At the cooling time, the cooker is ready to serve the porridge with crushed cinnamon as the topping.

50. Sweet Potato with Black Bean

What we need:

- 1 cup chopped onion
- 3 cups diced sweet potatoes
- 2 minced garlic cloves
- 2 cups boiled and dry black beans
- 2 tsp. chili flex

Cooking Method:

1. Cook the diced onion for 3–4 minutes, turning it brown.
2. Measure the garlic and stew until infused.
3. Mix the sweet potatoes and chili flex.
4. Course in the gravy and provide a final fuss before shutting the cover.
5. Count the ebony beans and scallions, and cook everything.
6. Season with salt and better chili flex if predicted.

51.   Walnut Duck

What we need:

- 1 cup duck minced
- 1 cup chopped walnuts
- 2 cups dried cranberries
- ½ tbsp. cinnamon
- 2 cups of water
- 1 cup of sunflower seeds

Cooking Method:

1. I minced the duck legs.
2. Set the meat, salt, and water in the oven.
3. Close the cover.
4. Bake for 12 minutes over high heat.
5. While the meat will cook, and then release it quickly.
6. While the cooker is getting cold, open the cover.
7. Combination in the parched seeds, nuts, cinnamon, cranberries, and sweetener.

52.   Mixed Berries and Granola

What we need:

- Honey 1 tbsp.
- 2 packs fresh acai puree (unsweetened)
- ¼ cup unsweetened any milk
- ½ cup mixed berries

Toppings:

- Shredded coconut
- Drizzle of honey
- Granola
- Mixed berries
- Sliced fresh fruit (such as banana, strawberries)
- Chia seeds

Cooking Method:

1. Blend fresh acai puree, berries, honey, milk, and ripe banana.

2. Grand until creamy and smooth, adding almond milk as required. Serve the acai smoothie in bowls.

3. Top acai smoothie bowls with your favorite ingredients.

4. Serve the Superfood Acai Bowl with Mixed Berries and Granola immediately for a healthy breakfast or snack!

53. Cottage Cheese and Fruit Bowl

What we need:

- 1 cup of mixed fresh fruits, like berries, diced melons, sliced bananas, or your favorite seasonal fruits

- 1 cup of cottage cheese

- Fresh mint leaves for garnish

- 1 tbsp. of honey

- A sprinkle of cinnamon

- 2 tbsp. of diced nuts (such as walnuts, almonds, or pistachios)

Cooking Method:

1. Start with fruit. Thoroughly wash and dry. Add bite-sized fruits to your plate.

2. Imagine the wonderful blend of fresh fruit hues and scents.

3. Scoop cottage cheese gently onto a dish to settle its creamy texture.

4. Smooth cottage cheese is pleasant.

5. Cottage cheese with fruit is great. For beauty, use a color combination.

6. Imagine the exhilaration each bite will bring from the texture and flavor contrast.

7. With a tbsp. of honey, sweeten cottage cheese and strawberries. Sprinkle cinnamon for flavor and heat.

8. Top it with chopped nuts. Crispy texture complements creamy cottage cheese and juicy fruits.

9. This dish is creamy, juicy, and crunchy.

10. Add fresh mint to cottage cheese and berries. Greenery will enhance the feast.

11. Enjoy every bite of this Cottage Cheese and Fruit Bowl's creamy cottage cheese, sweet fruits, and crunchy nuts. Mix ingredients for flavor explosion or diversity.

12. Relax and enjoy this nutritious, creamy, and fruity bowl.

54.   Apple Cinnamon Baked Oatmeal

What we need:

- 1 tsp. of powdered cinnamon
- 2 tbsp. of honey
- 4 cups of oats
- 2 medium-sized apples, diced
- 1/4 cup of raisins or dried cranberries
- 1 3/4 cups of milk
- For the oatmeal, 1 tsp. of baking powder rises and becomes fluffy.
- ½ cup minced nuts
- 1/4 tsp. of salt to enhance the overall taste
- 1 tsp. vanilla extract
- One large egg

Cooking Method:

1. Rolling oats, sliced apples, chopped almonds, raisins or dried cranberries, maple syrup (or honey), cinnamon, salt, and pure baking powder should be mixed. Add cinnamon and mix well.

2. Enjoy the bowl's tastes and textures.

3. Take another dish; mix the vanilla, milk, and egg. Mix the gravy and dry ingredients. Cover the dry elements with milk. Rich oatmeal batter.

4. Level the oatmeal batter pan. Consider oatmeal's beauty and oven changes. Bake or microwave the dish or pan for 30–35 minutes to light brown the top and set the oats.

5. Bake and smell oats at home. Cool the oats perfectly after baking. Add almonds, maple syrup, Greek yogurt, or apples to Apple Cinnamon Baked Oatmeal.

6. People might enjoy warm-cooked oats in considerable amounts for their calming tastes and textures. The first mouthful reveals delicious apples, cinnamon, and chewy oats. Let your taste buds dance.

7. In a sealed fridge, it lasts three days. Change it up by serving it cold or microwave.

55. Coconut Mango Chia Pudding

What we need:

- 2 cups of coconut milk
- Peel and dice one ripe mango.
- 1/4 cup chia seeds
- 1 tbsp. of maple syrup for natural sweetness
- For a hint of aromatic warmth,
- Add ½ tsp. Vanilla essence.
- Fresh mint leaves

Cooking Method:

1. Blend coconut milk, chia seeds, mango, vanilla, and maple syrup. Enjoy mango slices' brilliant color and coconut milk's scent.

2. To uniformly distribute and submerge chia seeds, forcefully stir coconut milk. After the water absorbs for 5 minutes, the chia seeds gel.

3. Chia seeds thicken the pudding, making it creamy and delicious. Whisk the mixture after 5 minutes to disperse the chia seeds.

4. To harden and taste, cover and chill the bowl for 2 hours or overnight.

5. As the pudding cools, flavors blend and chia seeds soften. Let the pudding set before gently combining.

6. Use glasses or plates to serve the scrumptious mango coconut chia pudding. For visual appeal, sprinkle fresh mint leaves on each dish.

7. Each scoop of chilled mango coconut chia pudding has tropical tastes and a creamy texture.

56. Vegetable Rice

What we need:

- ½ cup split yellow mung dal
- ½ cup basmati rice
- ½ tsp. turmeric powder
- Mixed vegetables (e.g., carrots, peas, zucchini)
- Ghee or oil for cooking
- A tsp. of asafoetida (hing)

- ½ tsp. cumin seeds
- Salt to taste
- Cilantro leaves for decorate

Cooking method:

1. After being washed and separated for around half an hour, the rice and mung dal may be soaked.

2. Put some ghee or oil on to simmer in a saucepan, then sprinkle in some cumin seeds and watch them pop.

3. After a few minutes of cooking, sprinkle in some asafoetida, some powdered turmeric, and a mixture of veggies.

4. After draining the rice and mung dal, place them in the saucepan and give them a quick sauté.

5. Put in some water, cover it, and let it simmer until it's done.

6. Salt should be added, and cilantro should be used as a garnish. Vegetable Rice is a dish that consists of vegetables and should be served.

57.   Meat with asparagus

What we need:

For the meat base:

- 600 g of brown rice
- 3 tbsp of cumin oil
- Chicken or vegetable stock
- Wine (optional)
- 1 onion, peeled and finely diced

For the vegetables:

- olive oil
- 4 cups vegetable stock
- trimmed asparagus 2 bunches
- 2 bunches of fresh basil, leaves chopped
- Coconut oil
- Salt
- black pepper

- sap and Zest of 2 lemons

Cooking method:

1. Add flavor to brown rice by cooking it in chicken or vegetable stock instead of water. Heat cumin oil in a big pan on medium.

2. Add chopped onion and sauté until transparent. Stir the sautéed onion into the cooked rice. Optional wine splash. Set aside.

3. In a separate pan, boil 4 cups chicken or vegetable stock. Add trimmed asparagus and cook 3–4 minutes until tender-crisp. Drain and set aside.

4. A small amount of coconut oil should be heated in a skillet over medium heat. Add cooked asparagus and sauté 1-2 minutes.

5. Season with lemon zest, juice, and salt. Stir well. Chop basil and add to asparagus. Mix thoroughly.

6. Use plates to base the rice mixture. Put asparagus and basil on top. Add extra virgin avocado or olive oil.

7. Add freshly ground black pepper to taste.

8. This tasty and healthy meal is best served immediately.

58.   Chickpea and Spinach Curry

What we need:

- 1 cup cooked chickpeas
- 1 onion, minced
- Coriander paste 1 tsp.
- 2 cups of fresh spinach leaves
- 1 tomato, cubed
- 1 tsp. garlic paste
- Grated ginger 1 tsp.
- A tsp. of cumin paste
- Ghee or oil for cooking
- Cilantro leaves for decorate
- Salt to taste

Cooking method:

1. While the ghee or oil is heating up in the cooker, put the chopped garlic, ginger, and onion. Fry until they becomes transparent.

2. Mix in some coriander powder and cumin, as well as some diced tomatoes. Cook the tomato until it becomes more pliable.

3. Add chickpeas that have been cooked and fresh spinach leaves. Cook the spinach until it becomes limp.

4. Add some salt to taste, and then finish it off with some cilantro leaves. Serve up this bean and spinach stew that is filled with protein.

59. Quinoa Salad with Lemon-Tahini Dressing

What we need:

- Cucumber slices
- Cherry tomatoes, cut into half
- Mixed salad greens
- 1 cup boiled quinoa
- 2 onion slices
- ¼ cup toasted sunflower seeds
- Fresh mint leaves for decorate

For the lemon-tahini decorating:

- 1 clove minced garlic
- 2 tbsp. of lime sap
- 3 tbsp. tahini
- Salt-pepper to taste
- A drizzle of olive oil

Cooking method:

1. Mix quinoa that has been cooked, assorted salad vegetables, onion slices, tomatoes, cucumber, tomatoes, and roasted sunflower seeds in a big bowl.

2. To create the dressing, put the tahini, lemon Sap, garlic minced and salt-pepper into a separate dish and combine all of the ingredients together.

3. After drizzling the coating over the salad, toss it to evenly cover the ingredients.

4. This energizing quinoa salad would be perfect with some fresh mint leaves sprinkled on top.

60.   Lentil

What we need:

- 1 cup split yellow mung dal
- 4 cups of water
- Mixed vegetables (e.g., carrots, peas, spinach)
- ½ tsp. turmeric powder
- A tsp. of cumin seeds
- Ghee or oil for cooking
- Salt to taste
- Fresh coriander leaves for decorate
- A tsp. of asafoetida (hing)

Cooking method:

1. It is necessary to wash the mung dal and then soak it for close to half an hour.
2. The cumin seeds and the substance should be added after the ghee or oil has been prepared.
3. After a few minutes of sautéing, add the pre-cut vegetable mix.
4. After being allowed to soak, the mung dal needed to be rinsed and then transferred to the pan along with the water.
5. Cook the dal in the turmeric powder for a sufficient amount of time until it is soft.
6. Add some salt, and then garnish with some fresh coriander that has been chopped. The lentil soup ought to have been offered since it would calm you down.

61.   Quinoa and Vegetable Stir-Fry

What we need:

- Fresh ginger paste 1 tsp.
- Ghee or oil for cooking
- Salt-pepper to taste
- 1 tsp. garlic paste
- Mixed stir-fry vegetables
- Cumin paste 1 tsp.
- A little bite of crushed coriander

- A tsp. of turmeric powder
- 1 cup cooked quinoa
- Fresh basil leaves for decorate

Cooking method:

1. Take a cooker; melt the ghee, and then put the garlic, cut finely, and the grated ginger. To quickly sauté in oil.

2. Add a stir-fry vegetable mix and continue cooking until the veggies are crisp-tender.

3. Combine the cumin paste seeds, powdered coriander seeds, and turmeric powder in a bowl by stirring them together.

4. After adding the cooked quinoa, mix everything together to incorporate.

5. Add a little Salt-pepper before serving.

6. Savor every bite of this Quinoa and Vegetable Stir-Fry, which is garnished with fresh basil leaves.

62.   Stuffed Bell Peppers

What we need:

- Salt to taste
- 1 cup boiled mung dal
- 1 cup Bell peppers (choose your preferred color)
- A tsp. of cumin paste
- 1 cup Mixed vegetables (e.g., zucchini, corn, peas)
- Cilantro leaves for decorate
- A tsp. of coriander powder
- brown rice that has been cooked

Cooking method:

1. Blanch the peppers in water that has been brought to a boil for a few minutes.

2. Warm the ghee in a separate pan, then add the rice, the mixed vegetables, and either the mung dal or the beans that have been prepared. To mix everything together, stir.

3. Mix in the roasted cumin, powdered coriander, and salt until evenly distributed.

4. Bake the stuffed bell peppers for a sufficient amount of time to ensure that the peppers become soft.

5. Serve these seasoned stuffed bell peppers with some cilantro as a garnish.

63.   Chickpea and Vegetable Curry

What we need:

- finely chopped 1 onion
- 1 tsp.   garlic paste
- 1 cup cooked chickpeas
- A tsp.   of grated ginger
- A tsp.   of cumin paste
- 1 tomato, chopped
- Cilantro leaves for decorate
- A tsp.   of turmeric powder
- 1 cup sliced Mixed vegetables (e.g., carrots, cauliflower, green beans)
- Salt to taste
- A tsp.   of coriander powder
- Ghee or oil for cooking

Cooking method:

1. While the ghee or oil is heating up in the pan, add the ginger, garlic, and onion that have been diced. Cook until the aromas develop.

2. After adding the mixed veggies, continue to cook them until they start to become tendered.

3. Combine the roasted cumin, crushed coriander, and turmeric powder by stirring them together.

4. Add chopped tomatoes and chickpeas that have already been cooked. Cook the tomato until it becomes more pliable.

5. Add some salt to taste, and then finish with some cilantro on top. Serve this satisfying curry made with chickpeas and vegetables.

64. Spinach and Tofu Salad

What we need:

- Cubed firm tofu
- Fresh spinach leaves
- Sliced cucumbers
- Cherry tomatoes, halved
- A handful of roasted pumpkin seeds
- Fresh mint leaves for decorate
- Sliced red onions

For the lemon-tahini dressing:

- Salt-pepper to taste
- 2 tbsp. tahini
- Sap of 1 lemon
- 1 tsp. garlic paste
- butter

Cooking method:

1. Fresh spinach leaves, cubed tofu, cherry tomatoes, cucumber slices, red onion slices, and roasted pumpkin seeds should be mixed together in a big dish before serving.

2. To create the dressing, put the tahini, lemon zest, garlic minced and pepper-salt into a separate dish and mix the entire element together.

3. After sprinkling the sauce over the salad, toss it to evenly cover the ingredients.

4. Enjoy this refreshing and nourishing   salad made with spinach and tofu, which you can finish with fresh mint leaves.

65.   Lentil and Vegetable Stir-Fry

What we need:

- Mixed stir-fry vegetables (e.g., bell peppers, snap peas, carrots)
- 1 cup cooked red or brown lentils
- ¼ tsp. of cumin paste
- ½ tsp. turmeric powder
- Salt-pepper to taste

- Ghee or oil for cooking
- A tsp. of coriander powder
- Fresh basil leaves for decorate

Cooking method:

1. 1. Start by melting the ghee or oil in a pan, then adding the stir-fry vegetables and cooking them over medium heat until they are crisp-tender.
2. Mix in some coriander powder, cumin, and turmeric, as well as some cumin paste.
3. After adding the cooked lentils, mix everything together to incorporate.
4. Add a little Salt-pepper before serving.
5. Savor this nourishing lentil and vegetable stir-fry, which is garnished with fresh basil leaves and served with brown rice.

66.   Quinoa and Lentil Pilaf

What we need:

- ½ tsp. cumin paste
- 1 cup cooked quinoa
- Sautéed mixed vegetables (e.g., bell peppers, broccoli, peas)
- Salt, pepper
- ½ cup cooked red or brown lentils
- A bite of turmeric powder
- A tsp. of minced coriander
- Ghee
- parsley leaves for decorate

Cooking method:

1. Warm the ghee in a cooker, and then put the sautéed mixed veggies plus continue stirring so that the vegetables are fragrant.
2. Combine the cumin paste, powdered coriander, and ginger paste by stirring them together.
3. Toss the quinoa and lentils together once they have been cooked.
4. Add a little Salt-pepper before serving.
5. Served with crisp parsley leaves for decorate.

67.   Vegetable Upma

What we need:

- 1 cup semolina (suji or rava)
- 2 tbsp. oil or ghee
- ½ tsp. mustard seeds
- ¼ cup slice mixed vegetables (e.g., carrots, peas)
- A few curry leaves
- Salt to taste
- ¼ tsp. turmeric powder

Cooking method:

1. Bring ghee or oil to a low simmer in a skillet and add cumin seeds and mustard seeds.
2. Add the chopped vegetables to the pan and keep cooking them till the veggies are just starting to get tender. Mix in the semolina, and then roast the mixture until it is a golden brown color.
3. Stir in the curry powder, salt, and curry leaves.
4. Add the hot water while continuing to whisk the mixture to prevent lumps from forming.
5. Place a lid on the pan and continue to cook the upma over a low flame for a few minutes, until it is fluffy and fully cooked.
6. Top with chopped cilantro and serve immediately.

68.   Rice Pudding

What we need:

- ½ cup basmati rice
- 4 cups milk (dairy or non-dairy)
- ¼ cup jiggery or brown sugar
- ¼ tsp. grated cardamom
- Chopped pistachios and almonds for garnish
- A few saffron threads (optional)

Cooking method:

1. After it has been washed and let to soak for a quarter of an hour.

2. Once the rice has been steeped for the appropriate amount of time, transfer it to a large saucepan while bringing the milk to a boil.

3. Continue to cook over low heat, stirring the mixture regularly, till the rice is completely soft and the sauce has set.

4. Mix in the powdered cardamom, jiggery or brown sugar, and the threads of saffron (if you're using them).

5. Pistachios and almonds, chopped, should be sprinkled over top.

6. You may serve it warm or cold, whichever you want better.

69.   Spiced Oats

What we need:

- rolled oats ½ cup

- 2 cups of water

- Grated cinnamon ¼ tsp.

- ¼ tsp. grated cardamom

- A tsp. of ginger paste

- Chopped dates or figs for sweetness

- Chopped pistachios or almonds for garnish

Cooking method:

1. The rolled oats should be added to water that has been brought to a boil in a saucepan.

2. Mix in some ginger paste, some ground cinnamon, and some grated cardamom. Stir well.

3. Cook the oats until they have reached the desired consistency and are fully cooked.

4. For a touch of natural sweetness, try incorporating some chopped figs or dates.

5. Pistachios or almonds, diced, may be used as a garnish for dishes to add crunch and taste.

70.   Broken Wheat Porridge

What we need:

- Ground fennel seeds ¼ tsp.

- ½ cup broken wheat (daliya)

- 2 cups of water

- A tsp. of saffron threads (optional)

- Chopped dates or raisins for sweetness
- A drizzle of ghee (optional)

Cooking method:

1. Gently roast the broken wheat in the saucepan until it reaches a color similar to golden brown.

2. Fennel seeds that have been pulverized and saffron threads, if used, should be added to water.

3. Maintain the simmering temperature until the broken wheat is pliable and the sauce has thickened.

4. To get a natural sweetness, stir in some chopped dates or raisins.

DINNER

71.   Green Soup

What we need:

- 1 head of cauliflower, chopped
- 1 head of broccoli, chopped
- 1 small onion, chopped
- 2 cloves of minced garlic
- 4 cups of vegetable or chicken broth
- ½ cup heavy cream
- 2 tbsp. of olive oil
- Black pepper and salt to taste
- Fresh chives or parsley, for garnish (optional)

Cooking Method:

1. Dice the broccoli and cauliflower into small pieces. The olive oil should be heated in a large cooker over high heat.

2. Sauté the vegetables for two to three minutes, so that they release a fragrant aroma and become open and forthcoming. The florets of cauliflower and broccoli should be added to the saucepan. Stir them in with the sautéed onion and garlic, and keep cooking for two or three minutes more.

3. Transfer the chicken soup to cover the vegetables. If needed, add a bit more broth to ensure the vegetables are submerged.

4. Stir the ingredients all the way up to boiling, and then turn the heat into steam. The cauliflower and broccoli should be cooked for around fifteen to twenty minutes with the lid on the pot before they are soft and can be readily punctured with a fork.

5. Make use of a blender to mix everything together until it is silky smooth and creamy. If you were using a blender, put the soup that has been puréed back into the cooker.

6. Swirl in the heavy cream to add extra creaminess to the soup. Season it with black pepper and salt, to taste.

7. Warm the soup above simmering, whisking it from time to time, while it is at the desired temperature. Add the cream slowly so as not to boil. Ladle the warm cauliflower and broccoli soup into soup dishes. If you wish, decorate with minced fresh chives for a pop of flavor and color.

8. Serve this comforting and nutritious soup as a starter or a light meal. It's creamy, satisfying, and packed with the goodness of cauliflower and broccoli.

72. Sweet Potato and Chickpea Curry

What we need:

- Two sweet potatoes, cubed
- Cumin crushed 1 tsp.
- 1 onion, minced
- 2 cups cooked chickpeas
- A tsp. of crushed coriander
- 1 tsp. garlic paste
- 1 tomato, diced
- Fresh and crushed ginger 1 tsp.
- Ghee or oil for cooking
- Cilantro leaves for decorate
- Salt-pepper

Cooking method:

1. While the ghee or oil is heating up in the pan, add the ginger, garlic, and onion that have been diced. Cook until the aroma is released.

2. After adding the sweet potato cubes, continue cooking until they have become somewhat softer.

3. Combine the crushed cumin, powdered coriander, and grounded turmeric by stirring them together.

4. Add chopped tomatoes and chickpeas that have already been cooked. Cook the tomato until it becomes more pliable.

5. Add a little Salt-pepper before serving.

6. Serve this substantial sweet potato and chickpea stew with cilantro leaves as a garnish.

73.   Spaghetti Squash with Pesto

What we need:

- 1 spaghetti squash, halved and seeds removed
- Salt-pepper to taste
- Fresh pesto sauce
- Fresh basil leaves for decorate
- Cherry tomatoes, halved

Cooking method:

1. Bake the halves of the spaghetti squash until the flesh is soft and can be easily shredded into "spaghetti" strings.

2. Spaghetti squash should be tossed with fresh pesto sauce and cherry tomatoes before being seasoned with Salt-pepper.

3. For a lovely twist on spaghetti squash with pesto, top each serving with some fresh basil leaves.

74.   Red Lentil and Vegetable Soup

What we need:

- Mixed vegetables (e.g., carrots, celery, bell peppers)
- 1 cup of red lentils
- Pepper and Salt to taste
- 2 cloves diced garlic
- 1 onion, diced
- 1 pinch of cumin powder
- 1 tsp. of minced coriander
- A pinch of turmeric powder

- Fresh parsley leaves for decorate
- Ghee or oil for cooking

Cooking method:

1. The red lentils should be washed and then left aside.

2. Warm up some ghee in a saucepan, and then whisk in some minced garlic and onion. Fry so that the aroma is released.

3. After adding the mixed veggies, continue to cook them until they start to become tendered.

4. Combine the roasted cumin, coriander powder seeds, and turmeric powder by stirring them   together.
   The red lentils should be added, along with water to fully coat them.

5. Stir periodically over low heat until lentils thicken and soup is tender.

6. Add a little Salt-pepper before serving.

75. Quinoa and Vegetable Stir-Fry

What we need:

- Ghee or oil for cooking
- Fresh ginger powder 1 tsp.
- Salt to taste
- Minced 1 clove garlic
- Mixed stir-fry vegetables
- Cumin paste 1 tsp.
- A little bite of crushed coriander
- A tsp. of turmeric powder
- 1 cup cooked quinoa
- Fresh basil leaves for decorate

Cooking method:

1. Melt ghee or oil in a pan, add finely chopped garlic, and grated ginger. Quick oil sauté.

2. Add a stir-fry vegetable mix and continue cooking until the veggies are crisp-tender.

3. Combine the cumin paste seeds, powdered coriander seeds, and turmeric powder in a bowl by stirring them together.

4. After adding the cooked quinoa, mix everything together to incorporate.

5. Add a little Salt-pepper before serving.

6. Savor every bite of this Quinoa and Vegetable Stir-Fry, which is garnished with fresh basil leaves.

76. Stuffed Bell Peppers

What we need:

- Salt to taste
- 1 cup boiled brown rice
- 1 cup boiled chickpeas or mung dal
- 1 cup Bell peppers (choose your preferred color)
- A tsp. of cumin paste
- 1 cup Mixed vegetables (e.g., zucchini, corn, peas)
- Cilantro leaves for decorate
- A tsp. of coriander powder

Cooking method:

6. Remove the stems and seeds from the bell peppers, and then blanch the peppers in water that has been brought to a boil for a few minutes.

7. Melt the ghee or oil in a separate pan, then add the brown rice that has been cooked, the mixed vegetables, and either the mung dal or the beans that have been prepared. To mix everything together, stir.

8. Mix in the roasted cumin, powdered coriander, and salt until evenly distributed.

9. Bake the stuffed bell peppers for a sufficient amount of time to ensure that the peppers become soft.

10. Serve these stuffed bell peppers with some cilantro as a garnish.

77. Zucchini Noodles with Pesto

What we need:

- Zucchini, spiralizer into noodles
- Fresh pesto sauce
- Cherry tomatoes, halved
- Sliced black olives
- Fresh basil leaves for decorate

- Salt-pepper to taste

Cooking method:

1. It is recommended that the zucchini noodles be cooked in a pan until they become noticeably tendered.

2. In a bowl, mix the zucchini noodles, cherry tomatoes, and shaved black olives. Then, add the fresh pesto sauce and mix everything together.

3. A little salt and pepper should be sprinkled over the food before serving.

4. The addition of fresh basil leaves elevates the flavor of the invigorating   zucchini noodles with basil that are served.

78. Rice and Vegetable Pilaf

What we need:

- Sautéed mixed vegetables (e.g., carrots, peas, corn)
- 1 cup cooked basmati rice
- Salt to taste
- Chopped cashews or almonds
- A tsp. of grated cardamom
- Fresh mint leaves for decorate
- ¼ cup raisins or currants
- A tsp. of ground cinnamon
- Ghee or oil for cooking

Cooking method:

1. When the ghee or oil is hot, add the chopped cashews, almonds, and currants and stir to combine. Then add the sautéed mixed veggies.

2. Mix with some grated cardamom and cinnamon before serving.

3. Add the basmati rice that has been cooked, and mix everything together.

4. Add some salt to taste, and then finish it off with some fresh mint leaves. Take some time to savor the savory aroma of this Ayurvedic rice and veggie cushion.

79.   Chickpea and Quinoa Salad

What we need:

- 1 ½ cup cooked chickpeas
- Diced cucumbers
- 1 cup cooked quinoa
- Chopped fresh parsley
- Chopped red bell peppers
- Salt-pepper to taste
- A drizzle of lemon sap and olive oil

Cooking method:

1. Mix together in a bowl the quinoa that has been cooked, the chickpeas, the diced cucumber, the chopped red bell pepper, and the fresh parsley.

2. To provide a zesty taste, drizzle with a mixture of olive oil and lemon Sap.

3. Add a little Salt-pepper before serving. Take pleasure in this Ayurvedic chickpea and quinoa salad that is packed with nutrients.

80.   Cumin-Spiced Carrot Soup

What we need:

- Vegetable broth
- Salt-pepper to taste
- 1 onion, minced
- 4-5 large carrots, sliced
- A tsp. of grated ginger
- 2 minced garlic cloves
- Ghee or oil for cooking
- 1 tsp. cumin paste
- Cilantro leaves for decorate

Cooking method:

1. While the ghee or oil is heating up in the saucepan, add the ginger, garlic, and onion that have been diced. Cook until the aromas develop.

2. When they have reached the desired degree of tenderness, add sliced carrots to the pan.

3. Mix the cumin powder and swirl it in.

4. Cook the carrots for a sufficient amount of time for them to become soft, and then add enough veggie stock to cover them.

5. After everything has been blended to a smooth consistency, the soup should be seasoned with pepper and salt.

6. Add some cilantro leaves as a garnish. Experience the soothing effects of this Ayurvedic carrot soup flavored with cumin.

81.   Chickpea and Brown Rice Bowl

What we need:

- Ghee for cooking
- Boiled chickpeas 1 cup
- 1 cup boiled brown rice
- A tsp. of turmeric powder
- Fried mixed vegetables
- Crushed Coriander 1 tsp.
- Salt-pepper to taste
- Fresh basil leaves for decorate

Cooking method:

1. Beginning with a pan, melt the ghee or the oil, then add the sautéed mixed vegetables and continue cooking them until they are crisp-tender.

2. Mix in some coriander powder, cumin, and turmeric, as well as some cumin paste.

3. Toss the prepared brown rice and chickpeas together after adding them to the dish.

4. Before serving, season with a pinch of salt and pepper.

5. This chickpea and brown rice dish is Ayurvedic, so finish it off with some fresh basil leaves before you dig in.

82.   Nut and Fruit Oatmeal

What we need:

- 2 tbsp. of dehydrated fruit, such as cranberries, raisins, diced apricots, and diced apples
- ½ tsp. grated cinnamon A bit of salt
- ¾ cup of balled oats
- 2 tbsp. of diced nuts, like pecans or walnuts
- ½ cup refreshed berries

Cooking Method:

1. Boil oats in water in a cooker until they begin cooking. Decrease the flame and allow it to steam for approximately 4 minutes.

2. Count cinnamon and salt while mixing. Top with berries and fruits, and serve warm.

83.   Cabbage Porridge with Red Pesto

What we need:

- 1 cup of oats
- vegetable stock 3 cups
- Couscous 1 cup
- 1 tsp. of parched oregano
- 1 tbsp. of any pesto
- 1 cup of minced cabbage
- 1 cup of minced cherry tomatoes
- 1 tbsp. of seed
- Salt
- 1 tbsp. of linseed

Cooking Method:

1. Boil oats, couscous, pepper, oregano, salt, and vegetable broth in a little bowl on medium to low heat for approximately 5 minutes, mixing periodically.

2. Mix scallions, diced cabbage, and tomatoes when it becomes a smoothie. Mix in pesto and yeast.

3. Complete it with cherry tomatoes, linseeds, and pumpkin, and then serve it hot.

84. Tilapia Breaded

What we need:

- ½ tsp. nicely chopped garlic
- ½ tsp. paprika
- 1 cup coconut spread for breading
- 1 pepper
- salt
- 2 tilapia fillets, cutted into 3-inch stripes
- 2 egg whites beaten

Cooking Method:

1. Warm the cooker to 410°F.
2. Put a wire frame on a piece of cooking foil and cover it with coconut fat.
3. Blend coconut, pepper, garlic, paprika, and salt until well-combined. Try a surface dish.
4. Put the egg whites in another container.
5. Sink each portion of fish in the egg, and then cover all flanks and all the coconut breading mix.
6. They are standing on the ready-made frame.
7. Splash some dots of olive oil on each part. Fry until the fish is boiled through. The breading should be brown.
8. Serve with salad.

85. Roasted Butternut Squash Salad

What we need:

- Sliced red onions
- Cubed roasted butternut squash
- Toasted pumpkin seeds
- Fresh sage leaves for decorate
- Mixed salad greens
- Salt-pepper to taste
- A drizzle of balsamic vinaigrette dressing

Cooking method:

1. In a large bowl, mix cubed baked butternut squash with a variety of salad greens and sliced red onions.

2. For an extra crunch, sprinkle with pumpkin seeds that have been roasted.

3. Drizzle with a dressing made of balsamic vinegar and vinaigrette.

4. Serve this bright Ayurvedic Roasted Butternut Squash Salad with fresh sage leaves as a garnish, and then dig in!

86.　Cauliflower and Green Bean Stir-Fry

What we need:

- Green beans, trimmed and halved
- Fresh cauliflower florets
- A tsp. of ginger paste
- Ghee for cooking
- A tsp. of garlic paste
- A tsp. of cumin paste
- Sliced red bell peppers
- Salt and tamari or soy sauce for flavor
- Cilantro leaves for decorate

Cooking method:

1. Ghee or oil should be heated up in a pan. Include the florets from the cauliflower as well as the green beans. Sauté them until they reach the perfect texture of tender-crisp.

2. Add sliced red bell peppers and stir-fry until they soften.

3. Add the ginger paste, powdered garlic, and crushed cumin, and whisk to mix.

4. Flavor with tamari or soy sauce and salt for added more test.

5. Serve this Ayurvedic Cauliflower and Green Bean Stir-Fry with cilantro leaves for decorate and savor its delicious benefits.

87. Greek Salad with Quinoa

What we need:

- 1 cucumber, diced
- 1 cup cooked quinoa
- 1 red bell pepper, diced
- 1 cup cherry tomatoes, halved
- ½cup Kalamata olives, pitted and sliced
- ½red onion, thinly sliced
- Fresh oregano leaves for garnish
- ½cup crumbled feta cheese or tofu (for a vegan option)

Cooking method:

1. Mix together in a bowl the quinoa that has been cooked, the chopped cucumbers, the cherry tomatoes, the Kalamata olives, the diced red onions, and the feta cheese if you want it.

2. To make the dressing, place the dried oregano, lemon sap, pepper, and salt in a separate bowl, and then combine all of those ingredients together with the olive oil.

3. 3. Toss the salad after sprinkling the dressing over it and making sure all of the ingredients are uniformly coated.

4. Garnish with fresh oregano leaves and enjoy this Ayurvedic Greek Salad with Quinoa.

88. Turmeric-Spiced Lentil Salad

What we need:

For the Salad:

- ¼ cup roasted almonds, minced
- 1 cucumber, sliced
- 1 cup dried green or brown lentils, rinsed
- ½red onion, finely chopped
- 1 cup cherry tomatoes, cutted into half
- ¼ cup fresh mint, diced
- ¼ cup fresh cilantro, crushed
- ½cup crumbled pander or tofu (for a vegan option)

- 3 cups water

For the Turmeric Dressing:

- Black pepper to taste
- 1 tbsp. apple cider vinegar
- Olive oil 4 tbsp.
- Salt
- Cumin powder 1 tsp.
- Ground turmeric 1 tsp.
- 1 tsp. honey

Cooking method:

1. Brown lentils that have been cooked, carrots and celery that have been chopped and red bell peppers that have been diced should be combined in a dish.

2. In a separate bowl, blend the dressing ingredients (olive oil, lemon juice, garlic, turmeric powder, and other spices) until combined.

3. After adding the combination to the salad, swirls it well to ensure level coverage.

4. Savor this Ayurvedic lentil salad with turmeric and curry spice, and garnish it with some fresh parsley leaves.

89.   Mung Bean Stew

What we need:

- 1 cup whole green mung beans, soaked overnight
- 1 tsp. mustard seeds
- 2 tbsp. ghee or coconut oil
- 4 cups water
- 1 tsp. cumin seeds
- 2 tomatoes, cubed
- 1 onion, finely chopped
- 1 zucchini, cubed
- 1 carrot, cubed
- 1 tsp. ground turmeric
- 1 cup spinach, cubed

- ½ tsp. cayenne pepper (adjust to taste)
- 1 tsp. coriander powder
- Fresh cilantro for garnish
- Salt to taste

Cooking method:

1. Wash and rinse the mung beans, and soak for about 30 minutes.

2. While the ghee or oil is heating up in the saucepan, add the ginger, garlic, and onion that have been diced. Cook until the aromas develop.

3. After adding the mixed veggies, continue to cook them until they start to become tendered.

4. Combine the cumin paste, coriander powder, and turmeric powder by stirring them together.

5. After soaking, rinse mung beans and cover with water in a saucepan. Let the stew simmer until the beans are soft and thickened.

6. Add some salt to taste, and then finish it off with some cilantro leaves. Take some time to nurture your body with this Ayurvedic Mung Bean Stew.

90.   Quinoa and Vegetable Curry

What we need:

- 1 ½ cups boiled quinoa
- Mixed vegetables 1 cup
- 1 tsp. of powdered turmeric
- 1 minced, chopped
- 1 tsp. cumin paste
- 3 minced garlic cloves
- Grated ginger 1 tsp.
- Salt to taste
- Fresh basil leaves for decorate
- Ghee or oil for cooking

Cooking method:

1. While the ghee or oil is heating up in the pan, add the ginger, garlic, and onion that have been diced. Cook until the aromas develop.

2. After adding the mixed veggies, continue to cook them until they start to become tendered.

3. Combine the roasted cumin, coriander powder, and turmeric powder by stirring them together.

4. After adding the cooked quinoa, mix everything together to incorporate.

5. Before serving, add salt and top with basil leaves. Devour this nourishing

6. Ayurvedic curry made with quinoa and vegetables

91. Sweet Potato and Chickpea Bake

What we need:

- 3 sweet potatoes, skinned and cut into cubed
- 1 can chickpeas
- 3 tbsp. ghee
- Thinly sliced 1 red onion
- 1 tsp. cumin powder
- Cinnamon ½ tsp.
- Smoked paprika ½ tsp.
- Fresh cilantro for garnish
- Black pepper and salt to taste

Cooking method:

1. In the bottom of a baking dish, layer sweet potatoes, chickpeas, and finely chopped red onions.

2. Garlic that has been minced, cumin that has been ground, coriander that has been grated and turmeric that has been ground should be combined with ghee or oil in a separate bowl.

3. Using a drizzle, evenly distribute the spice mixture over the layers of sweet potato and chickpea.

4. Cook the sweet potatoes in the oven until they are cooked but still retain some of their crispiness.

5. Add some salt to taste, and then finish it off with some cilantro leaves. Devour this satisfying Ayurvedic casserole made with sweet potatoes and chickpeas.

92. Lentil and Spinach Dal

What we need:

- Fresh spinach leaves
- 1 cup red or brown lentils
- Minced 2 cloves of garlic
- 1 onion, slice
- 1 tsp. of grated fresh ginger
- 1 tsp. cumin powder
- A tsp. of crushed coriander
- Turmeric powder 1 tsp.
- Cilantro leaves for decorate
- Salt-pepper to taste
- Ghee for cooking

Cooking method:

1. After they have been washed, put the lentils aside.
2. While the ghee or oil is heating up in the saucepan, add the ginger, garlic, and onion that have been diced. Cook until the aroma is released.
3. Include fresh spinach and steam until wilted.
4. Mix in cumin paste, coriander powder, and turmeric powder.
5. The lentils should be covered with water at this point. Keep cooking over low heat till the lentils are mushy and the dal has thickened.
6. Before serving, season with a pinch of salt and pepper.
7. Enjoy this soothing Ayurvedic Lentil and Spinach Dal with some cilantro leaves sprinkled on top before digging in.

93. Vegetable and Tofu Stir-Fry

What we need:

- Mixed stir-fry vegetables
- Cubed firm tofu
- Ginger paste 1 tsp.
- Cumin paste 1 tsp.
- Sliced mushrooms
- A tsp. of minced garlic
- Ghee or oil for cooking
- Fresh basil leaves for decorate
- Salt and tamari or soy sauce for flavor

Cooking method:

1. In a pan, heat ghee or oil, add cubed tofu, and cook until it's lightly browned.
2. Add mixed stir-fry vegetables and sliced mushrooms, and sauté until they are tender-crisp.
3. Stir in ginger paste, garlic paste, and cumin paste.
4. Season with salt and tamari or soy sauce for flavor.
5. Garnish with fresh basil leaves and enjoy this protein-rich Ayurvedic vegetable and tofu stir-fry.

94. Quinoa and Roasted Vegetable Bowl

What we need:

- 1 cup cooked quinoa
- Roasted mixed vegetables (e.g., sweet potatoes, beets, and carrots)
- Sliced red onions
- A tsp. of turmeric powder
- Cumin paste 1 tsp.
- Coriander powder 1 tsp.
- Ghee or oil for cooking
- Fresh parsley leaves for decorate

- Salt-pepper to taste

Cooking method:

1. In a bowl, combine cooked quinoa, roasted mixed vegetables, and sliced red onions.

2. Stir in turmeric powder, cumin paste, and coriander powder.

3. Drizzle with ghee or oil for added flavor.

4. Season with Salt-pepper.

5. Garnish with fresh parsley leaves and savor this Ayurvedic Quinoa and Roasted Vegetable Bowl.

95. Chickpea and Vegetable Curry

What we need:

- 1 cup boiled chickpeas
- Mixed vegetables
- 1 minced onion
- 2 cloves of garlic finely minced
- A tsp. of crushed ginger
- Cumin paste 1 tsp.
- A tsp. of turmeric powder
- Ghee or oil for cooking
- Cilantro leaves for decorate
- Salt-pepper to taste

Cooking method:

1. In a pan, heat ghee or oil; add chopped onion, minced garlic, and grated ginger. Sauté until aromatic.

2. Add the mixed vegetables and cook until they begin to soften.

3. Stir in cumin paste, coriander powder, and turmeric powder.

4. Add the cooked chickpeas and simmer until well combined.

5. Season with Salt-pepper.

6. Garnish with cilantro leaves and enjoy this Ayurvedic chickpea and vegetable curry.

96. Roasted Portobello Mushrooms

What we need:

- Ground rosemary 1 tsp.
- Portobello mushrooms, cleaned and stemmed
- Sliced red onions
- Minced garlic
- Olive oil for cooking
- Fresh thyme leaves for decorate
- Salt to taste

Cooking method:

1. Take a baking dish, place the cleaned Portobello mushrooms and top with sliced red onions and minced garlic.
2. Sprinkle with ground thyme and ground rosemary.
3. Add a little olive oil, pepper, and salt to finish.
4. Roast the mushrooms in the oven for about 20 to 25 minutes, or until they are tender and wet, after placing them on a baking sheet.
5. Garnish with fresh thyme leaves and enjoy these aromatic Ayurvedic roasted Portobello mushrooms.

97. Lentil and Spinach-Stuffed Bell Peppers

What we need:

- Bell peppers (choose your preferred color)
- 1 cup cooked red or brown lentils
- Fresh spinach leaves
- Diced tomatoes
- A tsp. of coriander powder
- Chopped red onions
- A tsp. of paste cumin
- A tsp. of turmeric powder
- Ghee or oil for cooking
- Cilantro leaves for decorate

- Salt-pepper to taste

Cooking method:

1. Cut the tops off the bell peppers, remove the seeds, and blanch them in boiling water for a few minutes.

2. In a separate pan, heat ghee or oil, add chopped red onions, and sauté until translucent.

3. Add diced tomatoes and fresh spinach leaves, and cook until wilted.

4. Stir in cumin paste, coriander powder, and turmeric powder.

5. Mix in the cooked lentils, and season with Salt-pepper.

6. Stuff the bell peppers with this mixture and bake until the peppers are tender.

7. Garnish with cilantro leaves and enjoy these Ayurvedic lentils and spinach-stuffed bell peppers.

98.   Basmati Rice and Vegetable Pilaf

What we need:

- 1 cup cooked basmati rice
- Sautéed mixed vegetables (e.g., carrots, peas, corn)
- Chopped cashews or almonds
- A handful of raisins or currants
- A tsp. of grated cardamom
- Ghee or oil for cooking
- Fresh mint leaves for decorate
- Salt to taste

Cooking method:

1. In a pan, heat ghee or oil and add sautéed mixed vegetables, chopped cashews or almonds, and raisins or currants.

2. Stir in grated cardamom.

3. Add the cooked basmati rice and toss to combine.

4. Season with salt, and garnish with fresh mint leaves. Enjoy this fragrant Ayurvedic basmati rice and vegetable pillow.

99. Spiced Chickpea and Sweet Potato Curry

What we need:

- 1 onion, finely minced
- 1 cup cooked chickpeas
- 1 cup Sweet potatoes, diced
- 2 minced garlic cloves
- A tsp. of grated ginger
- 1 tsp. cumin paste
- Coriander powder 1 tsp.
- A pinch of turmeric powder
- Ghee or oil for cooking
- Cilantro leaves for decorate
- Salt-pepper to taste

Cooking method:

1. In a pan, heat ghee or oil; add chopped onion, minced garlic, and grated ginger. Sauté until aromatic.
2. Add sweet potatoes and cook until they start to soften.
3. Stir in cumin paste, coriander powder, and turmeric powder.
4. Add cooked chickpeas and simmer until the curry thickens and the sweet potatoes are tender.
5. Season with Salt-pepper.
6. Garnish with cilantro leaves and enjoy this comforting Ayurvedic chickpea and sweet potato curry.

100. Quinoa and Kale Salad

What we need:

- 1 cup cooked quinoa
- Fresh kale leaves, destemmed and chopped
- Cherry tomatoes, halved
- Sliced red onions
- Chopped almonds or walnuts

- A drizzle of olive oil and lemon Sap
- Salt-pepper to taste

Cooking method:

1. Mix chopped nuts, kale, cherry tomatoes, red onion, and cooked quinoa in a bowl.
2. Olive oil and fresh lemon juice provide a delicious finishing touch.
3. Add Pepper and salt to taste.
4. Get everything well combined by tossing the ingredients.
5. Try some of this Ayurvedic Quinoa and Kale Salad.

101. Eggplant and Chickpea Stir-Fry

What we need:

- 1 cup cooked chickpeas
- Cubed eggplant
- A tsp. of ginger paste
- Sliced red bell peppers
- A tsp. of cumin paste
- A tsp. of garlic paste
- Cilantro leaves for decorate
- Salt and tamari or soy sauce for flavor
- Ghee for cooking

Cooking method:

1. To make soft and slightly crispy eggplant, heat ghee or oil in a skillet and add cubed eggplant.
2. Stir-fry sliced red bell peppers until they soften, then add
3. Mix in the cumin paste, ginger paste, and garlic paste.
4. Stir in the chickpeas that have already been cooked.
5. To enhance the taste, sprinkle with salt and drizzle with tamari or soy sauce.
6. Serve this delicious Ayurvedic eggplant and chickpea stir-fry garnished with cilantro leaves.

102.   Mediterranean Stuffed Bell Peppers

What we need:

- Crumbled feta cheese (optional)
- Bell peppers (choose your preferred color)
- Diced cucumbers
- Cooked quinoa or brown rice
- Sliced Kalamata olives
- Fresh oregano leaves for decorate
- Chopped red onions

Cooking method:

1. Remove the stems and seeds from the bell peppers, and then blanch the peppers in water that has been brought to a boil for a few minutes.

2. Mix cooked quinoa or brown rice, minced cucumbers, Kalamata olives, chopped red onions, and feta cheese, if using, in a dish and keep aside.

3. Stuff the bell peppers with this mixture.

4. Bell peppers filled with Ayurvedic filling should be topped with fresh oregano leaves before serving. This dish takes its inspiration from the Mediterranean.

103.   Red Lentil and Vegetable Soup

What we need:

- Salt-pepper to taste
- 1 onion, minced
- 1 cup of red lentils
- Mixed vegetables (e.g., carrots, celery, peas)
- 3 minced garlic cloves
- A tsp. of coriander powder
- A tsp. of fresh grated ginger
- A tsp. of cumin paste
- A tsp. of turmeric powder
- Fresh parsley leaves for decorate
- Ghee for cooking

Cooking method:

1. Rinse the red lentils and set them aside.

2. While the ghee or oil is heating up in the saucepan, add the ginger, garlic, and onion that have been diced. Cook until the aroma is released.

3. After adding the mixed veggies, continue to cook them until they start to become tender.

4. Mix in the cumin paste, coriander that has been minced, and turmeric powder.

5. Cover the lentils with water. Stir periodically over low heat until lentils are cooked and soup thickens.

6. Before serving, season with a pinch of salt and pepper.

7. Serve this Ayurvedic Red Lentil and Vegetable Soup with a garnish of fresh parsley leaves, and do not forget the garnish!

104. Roasted Brussels sprouts with Mustard and Honey

What we need:

- 1 tsp. of Honey

- Brussels sprouts, trimmed and halved

- Lemon Sap 1 tsp.

- Mustard seeds 1 tsp.

- 2 tsp. of Olive oil

- Salt-pepper to taste

Cooking method:

1. Start by cutting the Brussels sprouts in half and placing them in a mixing bowl. Add honey and whole mustard seeds and mix.

2. Before putting them in the oven, they should be spread out in one layer on a baking sheet and arranged in the correct order.

3. They should be roasted in the oven for around 20–25 minutes, or until they are soft while maintaining their crispiness.

4. Season with pepper and salt, then sprinkle with lemon juice and finish with more salt and pepper.

5. Enjoy these Ayurvedic Roasted Brussels Sprouts with Mustard and Honey as a flavorful side dish.

DESSERT

105. Date and Nut Balls

What we need:

- Ghee or coconut oil
- Dates, pitted
- A tsp. of crushed nutmeg
- Mixed nuts (e.g., almonds, cashews, and walnuts)
- A tsp. of crushed cloves
- Grated cardamom

Cooking method:

1. Put the dates with the pits removed, the mixed nuts, the ghee or coconut oil, the shredded cardamom, the crushed nutmeg, and the crushed cloves into a grinder.
2. Continue to process the ingredients until they come together to create sticky dough.
3. Form the dough into a few balls using your hands.
4. You may choose to roll the balls in shredded coconut, but it's not required.
5. Put it in your fridge for approximately half an hour to get it nice and cold.
6. These Ayurvedic Date and Nut Balls are the perfect, delicious treat that will also give you a surge of energy.

106. Kheer

What we need:

- Milk or dairy-free milk
- Saffron threads
- Basmati rice
- Cardamom pods
- Ghee or coconut oil
- honey (for sweetness)
- Crushed pistachios and almonds for garnish

Cooking method:

1. After it has been rinsed, the rice should be soaked for half an hour in water.

2. In a saucepan, melt some ghee or coconut oil, and then sauté some cardamom pods until they release their aroma.

3. After draining the rice, add it to the cooking pot.

4. Mix with some milk and saffron strands.

5. Steam, stirring it often, until the rice is completely mushy and the pudding has thickened to the desired consistency.

6. Honey may be used to sweeten.

7. Pistachios and almonds, crushed, should be sprinkled over top.

8. Rich and fragrant, this Ayurvedic rice pudding is a delicious option for a sweet treat.

107. Coconut and Saffron Truffles

What we need:

- Almond flour
- Shredded coconut
- Honey (for sweetness)
- Saffron threads
- Chopped pistachios for garnish
- Ghee or coconut oil

Cooking method:

1. Shredded coconut, almond flour, saffron threads, ghee or coconut oil, honey,   should all be mixed together in a basin before proceeding.

2. Continue to blend the ingredients until they are cohesive and cohesively integrated.

3. Roll the dough into little balls, which should be around the size of truffles.

4. Cover each truffle with an additional layer of crushed coconut.

5. Pistachios, chopped, serve as a garnish for the dish.

6. Put it in the refrigerator for approximately half an hour to get it nice and cold.

7. As a decadent and satisfying dessert option, these Ayurvedic coconut and saffron truffles are a wonderful choice.

108. Spiced Poached Pears

What we need:

- Cardamom pods
- Ripe pears, peeled and halved
- Honey
- Water
- Cloves
- Cinnamon sticks

Cooking method:

1. Put the water, honey, and the spices (cinnamon sticks, cardamom pods, and cloves) in a saucepan and steam it.

2. After bringing the liquid up to a simmer, add the pears, which have been peeled and cut in half.

3. Cook the pears in a poaching liquid until they are soft and have taken on the flavor of the spices.

4. It may either be served warm or cooled.

5. Poached pears flavored with Ayurvedic spices make for a sweet treat that is both warm and aromatic.

109. Date and Almond Bliss Balls

What we need:

- Grated cardamom
- Dates, pitted
- A tsp. of crushed cloves
- Ghee or coconut oil
- Almonds
- A tsp. of crushed nutmeg

Cooking method:

1. Place dates that have had the pits removed, almonds, shredded cardamom, ghee or coconut oil, crushed nutmeg, and crushed cloves in the bowl of a grinder.

2. Continue to process the ingredients until they come together to create sticky dough.

3. Form bliss balls with the dough using your hands.

4. Put it in the refrigerator for approximately half an hour to get it nice and cold.

5. A delicious and wholesome dessert option, these Ayurvedic Date and Almond

6. Bliss Balls are made with dates and almonds.

110. Saffron and Rosewater Rice Pudding

What we need:

- Saffron threads
- Basmati rice
- Milk or dairy-free milk
- Ghee or coconut oil
- Rosewater
- Honey (for sweetness)
- Chopped pistachios and almonds for garnish

Cooking method:

1. After it has been rinsed, the rice should be soaked for half an hour in water.

2. When the ghee or coconut oil is hot, add the saffron threads and continue to cook them until the aroma is released.

3. After draining the rice, add it to the cooking pot.

4. After adding the milk, continue cooking the pudding over a low heat, stirring the mixture regularly, until the rice is soft and the pudding has thickened.

5. Honey may be used as a sweetener, and then a few drops of rosewater can be added.

6. Pistachios and chopped almonds should be sprinkled over top.

7. A fragrant and unique delicacy, this Ayurvedic saffron and rosewater rice

8. Pudding may be enjoyed as a sweet treat.

111. Almond and Cardamom Fudge

What we need:

- Ghee or coconut oil
- Almond butter
- Honey (for sweetness)
- Grated cardamom
- Chopped almonds for garnish

Cooking method:

1. In a bowl, combine almond butter, honey, crushed cardamom, ghee or coconut oil, and the sweetener of your choice, such as honey.

2. Combine all of the ingredients and stir them together well until the mixture reaches the consistency of fudge.

3. After pressing the mixture onto a tray, chopped almonds should be sprinkled on top after the tray has been smoothed out.

4. While you wait for it to set, you may chill it in the refrigerator to make it easier to handle.

5. These Ayurvedic almond and cardamom fudge bites are the ideal way to round off your dinner because of their decadent and nutty flavor.

112. Coconut and Cardamom Rice Cakes

What we need:

- Coconut milk
- Chopped pistachios for garnish
- Cooked rice
- Honey (for sweetness)
- Grated cardamom
- Ghee or coconut oil

Cooking method:

1. A bowl should be used for combining cooked rice, coconut milk, grated cardamom, ghee or coconut oil, honey, and mixing all of these ingredients together.

2. Make sure the ingredients are well combined.

3. Once pressing the mixture onto a tray, chopped pistachios should be sprinkled on top once the dough has been finished setting.

4. Put it in the refrigerator so that it can set up.

5. These Ayurvedic coconut and cardamom rice cakes are a fragrant and velvety treat that can be enjoyed by slicing them into squares and serving them. The cakes are flavored with cardamom and coconut.

113.   Chia-spiced poached apples

What we need:

- Water
- Apples, peeled and sliced
- Honey
- Chia spices (cinnamon, cloves, cardamom, and ginger)
- Chopped walnuts for garnish
- Ghee or coconut oil

Cooking method:

1. To make Chia, combine water, Chia spices, and a sweetener honey in a kettle.

2. After bringing the liquid up to a simmer, add the apples, which have been peeled and cut into thin slices.

3. The apples should be poached until they are tender and have taken on the flavor of the Chia spices.

4. You may serve this dish warm or cold and you can top it with chopped walnuts.

5. Poached apples with Chia spices are an Ayurvedic treat that will warm you up and satisfy your sweet tooth.

114.   Saffron and Pistachio Semolina Pudding

What we need:

- A pinch of Saffron threads
- 2 tbsp. of Ghee
- 1 cup of Semolina (suji)
- 1 cup of Honey   (for sweetness)
- 2 tbsp. of Chopped pistachios

Cooking method:

1. After heating the ghee, add the semolina to the pan.

2. Toast the semolina in the oven until it turns a golden color.

3. A sweetener such as honey, as well as saffron threads and chopped pistachios, should be added.

4. Continue to stir until the saffron has contributed its color and the semolina has been well covered.

5. To be served hot.

6. An aromatic and nutty dish, this Ayurvedic Saffron and Pistachio Semolina Pudding is made with semolina and saffron.

115. Chocolate Cheesecake

What we need:

- 1 tsp. vanilla
- ½ cup chocolate almond milk
- 2 cups of soaked cashews
- 2 tsp of softened olive oil
- 2 cups grated almonds
- flour 2 cups
- sugar 1 cup
- ½ cup vegan chocolate chips
- 1 cup of sugar

Cooking Method:

1. Combine the elements in the main index concurrently.

2. Shaking softly into the base of a 6-inch cake maker and 2- inches up the flanks.

3. Set it in the refrigerator while you assemble the stuffing.

4. Beat the dual-component index in a bowl until fluffy. Mix the grated coconut and blend.

5. Mix chocolate chunks and combine with a spoon for a nicely blended. Run the batter into the cake maker.

6. Place the dish in the oven, and then shut the cover.

7. Boil on a high flame for 50 minutes.

8. Stay 10 minutes back fast, removing stress.

9. Pull the pan gingerly and refrigerate it for two hours.

10. Roll the cakes in shredded coconut, crushed almonds, or cocoa powder, assuming they will have added consistency and explicit appeal. And ready to be enjoyed whenever a quick energy boost is needed.

116.   Banana Ice Cream

What we need:

- Four ripe bananas

- 2 tbsp. of almond butter

- ½ tsp. vanilla essence

- 1 tbsp. of honey

Cooking Method:

1. Peel the ripe bananas and slice them. Place the slices in a Ziploc bag or an airtight box and ice them for 2 hours until solid.

2. Once the bananas are prepared to dish up, extract the ice cream from the cooler and allow it to sit at normal temperature for a few moments to milden.

3. Transfer the set of banana slices to a mixer. Mix the almond butter, vanilla section, and honey.

4. Mix the combination quickly so the bananas break down and become pale. Rub down the flanks of the blender as needed.

5. Count any optional toppings, such as diced nuts, shredded coconut, chocolate chips, or fresh berries, if desired. Beat the blender a few times to combine the toppings.

6. Share the banana ice cream combination in a loaf pan or a freezer-safe receptacle. Smooth the top with a spatula.

7. Cover the receptacle and set it in the freezer for 1-2 hours, or until the ice cream is firm.

8. When prepared to dish up, extract the ice cream from the cooler and allow it to sit at a normal temperature for a few moments to milden.

117. Cherry Cake

What we need:

- Pie filling: cherry (20 oz.)
- Butter, unsalted (½ cup)
- Sour cream (1 cup)
- 2 cups of white flour
- Two eggs
- 1 tsp. vanilla
- Baking powder 1 tsp.
- Sugar

Cooking Method:

1. Dissolve the butter and heat the microwave to 350°F.
2. Finely mix the eggs, sour cream, butter, and vanilla in a small basin.
3. In another bowl, whisk together the flour and baking powder.
4. Later, combine the two mixtures, folding to mix thoroughly.
5. Grease your pan and pour the batter.
6. Expand the cherry mixture over the batter.
7. Bake them for around 40 minutes.

118. Saffron and Almond Semolina Pudding

What we need:

- 3 cups of Almond milk
- Semolina (suji) 1 cup
- 2 tbsp. of Ghee or coconut oil
- A pinch of Saffron threads
- Chopped almonds for garnish
- 1 cup of Honey (for sweetness)

Cooking method:

1. Ghee or coconut oil should be heated in a pan before adding semolina to it.
2. Toast the semolina in the oven until it turns a golden color.

3. Saffron threads and almond milk should be added.

4. Cook over a low heat, stirring the mixture on occasion, until the semolina is completely soft and the pudding has reached the desired consistency.

5. Honey or jiggery may be used to sweeten.

6. Almonds, chopped, serve as a garnish.

7. The Saffron and Almond Semolina Pudding is a dish that is both creamy and nutty, and it is delicious.

119.   Coconut and banana ice cream

What we need:

- 1 cup Coconut milk
- 1 Ripe bananas
- 2 tbsp. of Honey or jiggery (for sweetness)
- 2 tbsp. of Shredded coconut

Cooking method:

1. In a blender, combine ripe bananas, coconut milk, shredded coconut, and the sweetener of your choosing, whether it is honey or jiggery. Blend until smooth.

2. Mix until lumps are eliminated.

3. Combine everything in such a way that it becomes velvety smooth.

4. Put the mixture in a container, and then put the container with the mixture into the freezer. Leave it there until the mixture reaches the consistency of ice cream.

5. This Ayurvedic coconut and banana ice cream is a creamy dessert that can be served in scoops and eaten. It has a tropical flavor profile and is made with coconut and bananas.

120.   Carrot Halwa

What we need:

- 3 Grated carrots
- 3 tbsp. of Ghee or coconut oil
- A pinch of Grated cardamom
- 3 tbsp. of Chopped cashews and raisins
- 3 tbsp. of Honey (for sweetness)

Cooking method:

1. When the ghee or coconut oil has been heated up in the pan, grated carrots should be added to the mixture.

2. The carrots should be sautéed until they reach the desired degree of tenderness.

3. The cardamom should be grated, while the cashews and raisins should be chopped up into smaller pieces.

4. Continue to cook for a few more minutes, until the carrots have a golden color and the nuts have a scent similar to that of toasted nuts.

5. To sweeten, either honey or jiggery may be used.

6. A classic Ayurvedic dessert, carrot and cardamom Halwa has a flavor profile that is warm and nutty at the same time. To each his own!

121. Date and Walnut Delight

What we need:

- 1 cup pitted dates

- 1 cup walnuts

- 1 tbsp. coconut oil

- A pinch of ground cinnamon

- 2 tbsp. honey

Cooking method:

1. Make sure the dates have pits in them. If the walnuts aren't already broken up, do so now.

2. Pitted dates, walnuts, ghee or coconut oil, a pinch of cardamom, a pinch of ground cinnamon, and honey should all be put into a grinder.

3. Combine ingredients into a smooth, sticky dough. Shape little quantities of mixture into squares or balls with your hands.

4. Put the balls or squares that you've made on a tray that has been lined with parchment paper. To make them set, put them in the fridge for at least 30 minutes.

5. The Ayurvedic Date and Walnut Delight are ready to be served after it has been chilled. For an extra touch, you can roll the balls or pieces in shredded coconut if you want to.

6. Any food that is left over should be kept in the fridge in a container that won't let air in. Take a moment to enjoy this Ayurvedic treat by savoring its flavors as well as textures.

122. Spiced Coconut Rice Pudding

What we need:

- 2 cups coconut milk
- 1 cup Basmati rice
- 2 tbsp. ghee or coconut oil
- ½ tsp. ground cinnamon
- 1 tsp. ground cardamom
- Shredded coconut for garnish
- 3 tbsp. honey

Cooking method:

1. Run cold water over the basmati rice until the water is clear. Allow the rice to soak in water for 30 minutes.

2. Set ghee or coconut oil on medium heat in a pot. Take the rice out of the water and add it to the pot. Cook the rice for a few minutes until it's just barely toasted.

3. Pour in the coconut milk and mix it well. Bring the stuff together to a slow boil.

4. Turn down the heat, cover the pot, and let the rice cook slowly until it soaks up the coconut milk and gets soft. Add ground cinnamon and cardamom and mix them in to give the pudding a fragrant scent.

5. You can make the dessert sweeter by adding honey or sugar. Mix the sweetener well until it's all mixed in.

6. When the rice pudding gets smooth and creamy, take it off the heat. Add chopped coconut as a garnish to add more taste and texture.

7. Take a moment to enjoy this Ayurvedic Spiced Coconut Rice Pudding's rich coconut flavor and the mild heat of the spices. If you have food left over, put it in the fridge so you can enjoy it later.

123. Dark Chocolate-Covered Almonds

What we need:

- 1 cup unbroken almonds

- 8 ounces dark hard chocolate, chopped or in chip form

- Optional toppings: shredded coconut, sea salt, ground pretzels, parched fruit, or sprays

Cooking Method:

1. Roast them for 10 minutes to eliminate the spice and make them golden. Stir periodically to toast evenly.

2. Remove the almonds from the heat and cool. Make dark chocolate melt on a microwave-safe plate. Avoid overheating by melting chocolate in 30-second increments in the microwave and mixing well.

3. Take away the chocolate from the warmth and allow it chill. This prevents chocolate from over softening almonds. Cover a handful of almonds with dissolved chocolate. Lift the almonds from the chocolate with a knife or slotted scoop to drain excess chocolate.

4. Without touching, place chocolate-covered almonds on a parchment-lined baking sheet. This keeps them apart during solidification.

5. Sprinkle salt, shredded coconut, broken pretzels, or dried fruit on chocolate-covered almonds instead of chocolate. The design character and consistency will be unique. Repeat until the almonds are covered.

6. Set the chocolate-covered almonds at room temperature for an hour to firm and shine.

7. After the chocolate hardens, store dark chocolate-covered almonds in an airtight container or cosmetic gift box. Store them in darkness and cold.

124. Maple-Walnut Pots

What we need:

- ½ cup of unsweetened soy milk is required.

- ¼ tsp. of pure vanilla essence

- 1½ tsp. of plain gelatin

- ½ cup fat-free Greek yogurt with vanilla flavor

- ½ cup of fat-free or low-fat buttermilk

- ⅓ cup of pure maple syrup

- A speck of salt from the ocean

- A garnish of 2 tbsp. of chopped walnuts

Cooking Method:

1. Simmer soy milk, sugar, and vanilla in a small saucepan. Stir often while heating the mixture for two minutes over medium heat until it's just above room temperature.
2. Heat the mixture until it is boiling for three minutes after adding the gelatin.
3. Turn off the stove and let it cool for a little.
4. Whisk together all the ingredients except the walnuts after adding them.

125. Carrot Cookies with Chocolate Chip

What we need:

- ⅛ cup of applesauce that has not been sweetened

- 1 egg, big in size

- A quarter cup of shredded carrots

- 1/3 cup of almond meal

- A quarter of a cup of dairy-free dark-colored chocolate chips

- 1 milliliter of unadulterated maple syrup

- ¼ tsp. of the baking powder

- ½ tsp. of cinnamon powder

Cooking Method:

1. Turn up the microwave. Prepare a parchment paper lining for your baking sheet.

2. In an enormous combining bowl, whisk the almond nutrition, baking powder, chocolate chips, carrots, applesauce, maple syrup, eggs, as well as grated cinnamon. Combine all of the ingredients by stirring each other until the mixture takes on the texture of thick dough.

3. Place tbsp.-sized rounds onto the baking sheet that has been prepared. Bake the bread for ten to fifteen minutes, so that it begins to become a light brown color. Dish up.

126. Banana-Oatmeal Cookies

What we need:

- ¼ cup olive oil, plus additional oil for greasing
- ¾ cup unadulterated honey
- 1 egg
- 2 very big, perfectly ripe bananas, mashed.
- 2 tsp. of pure vanilla essence
- ½ cup of 100% whole wheat flour
- A half cup of almond flour
- A pinch of kosher salt
- ½ tsp of baking soda
- 3.0 ounces of rolled oats

Cooking Method:

1. Preheat oven to 375°F. Oil two rimmed baking sheets.
2. Whisk eggs, honey, and oil in a large basin. Add the bananas and stir well.
3. Mix all the flour, butter, and salt in a bowl. Mix the banana mixture with the flour. Mix in rolled oats.
4. Scoop tbsp.-sized rounds onto the prepared baking sheets. Roast cookies for ½ to ½ minutes, monitoring for fire in the last stages.
5. To serve.

127. Marinated Berries

What we need:

- 2 cups of fresh strawberries, which have been hulled and cut into quarters
- 1 cup of fresh blueberries, if you want them
- 1 tbsp. of natural honey
- A tbsp. worth of balsamic vinegar
- 1/8 tsp. pepper

Cooking Method:

1. Combine the strawberries, blueberries (if desired), honey, and cinnamon in a large bowl.

2. Combine the pepper, mint (if using it), and vinegar in a big basin that is not reactive.

3. Give the flavors some time to come together for no less than 25 minutes and up to 2 hours.

128.   Tofu Mocha Mousse

What we need:

- 4 ounces of dark chocolate with a percentage of 70%, cut very finely
- ½ cup of soy milk
- ½ tsp. of espresso powder
- ½ tsp. of pure vanilla essence
- A speck of salt from the ocean
- 4 ounces of silken tofu, well drained

Cooking Method:

1. Put the chocolate in the bowl that's about the size of your palm and set it aside.

2. Mix soy milk, coffee powder, vanilla extract, and salt in a small pot. Heat a pot on medium-high. Bring mixture to boil.

3. Bring the mixture to a boil, and then sprinkle it over the chocolate when it has cooked. After letting the mixture sit for ten minutes, whisk it until all of the ingredients are combined.

4. Add it to the tofu in your blender and mix until smooth. Process it in a blender until it is completely smooth.

5. The mixture should be divided into two bowls, covered, and refrigerated for at least two hours until firm. Serve up.

129.   Dessert Made with Grilled Mango

What we need:

- 1 mango, peeled, seeded, and cut to your preference
- 1 lime, sliced into eight equal-sized wedges

Cooking Method:

1. Position the oven rack so that it is in the top third of the oven, and preheat the oven and broiler. Use aluminum foil to line the bottom of your broiler pan.

2. Place the mango slices so that they are in a single layer in the pan that has been prepared—broil approximately eight to ten minutes, or until there are brown patches throughout.

3. Divide the mixture evenly between two dishes, then strain the lime wedges over the top and carry it out.

130. Date Brownies

What we need:

- 2 cups of dates with the pits removed
- 3 jumbo-sized eggs
- 1 standard cup of grated almonds
- ½ tsp. of cocoa powder
- A quarter cup of avocado oil
- One tsp. of baking soda
- A little bit of salt

Cooking Method:

1. Turn the oven on to preheat. Spray some oil in your 8-inch baking dish, and then grease it.

2. Place your small pan of water on the stove and increase the temperature to a high setting. Take the pan away from the heat immediately.

3. Once the pits have been removed from the dates, set them in a bowl, cover them with water in a separate pot, and start to boil. Let them soak for 15 minutes. Empty out.

4. Put the dates and the two tbsp. of water into your food processor and pulse until combined to make a smoothie consistency.

5. Mix the eggs one by one, mixing in between each addition of an egg.

6. Stirring the dry ingredients together will combine all of the ingredients. Bake for thirty minutes, or until the dish can be pierced all the way through with a toothpick made of stainless steel and comes out clean.

7. Take the dish out of the oven. After allowing it to cool, carve it into ¼ equal pieces. Dish up.

131. Yogurt and Berry Freezer Pops

What we need:

- 1 fluid ounce of either blueberries or blackberries that is fresh.
- ½ cup of Greek yogurt that is plain and nonfat.
- 2 tbsp. of natural honey
- 2 cups of low-fat milk

Cooking Method:

1. Put all of the ingredients into your blender and blitz them together until the combination is perfectly soft.

2. Remove the liquid to ice pop molds, and then store the molds in the freezer for at least six hours before serving.

132. Baked Halibut Steaks

What we need:

- 2 halibut steaks, each weighing five ounces
- ½ of a lemon, segmented and cut into wedges
- 1 tbsp. minced parsley
- 1 tbsp. of olive oil
- ¼ of a tsp. of grated black pepper

Cooking Method:

1. The temperature inside the oven has to be set to 350 degrees Fahrenheit. A piece of parchment paper should be placed on an oven rack before it is set aside.

2. Prepare a baking sheet for the halibut fillets by laying them out in one layer. Put some oil on the pinnacle of it, and next season it with pepper on both sides.

3. Bake for a total of six to eight minutes. After you have flipped the halibut, continue cooking it for another 5 minutes or until it can be easily flaked apart. Take the dish out of the oven.

4. Accompany the halibut with lemon slices and parsley on the serving plate.

133.   Chickpea Salad Sandwich

What we need:

- One drained and rinsed can of chickpeas with reduced salt content, which comes in a 15-ounce can
- ¼ cup of red onion that has been coarsely chopped
- ¼ cups of Greek yogurt that is unflavored, unsweetened, and low in fat
- ½ tsp. of mustard made from whole grains
- Black pepper, grated to the desired degree
- 4 pieces of bread made with healthy grains

Cooking Method:

1. Place the chickpeas in the basin and use a fork to mash them roughly, making sure to leave some intact for texture.

2. After adding the onion, garlic, mustard, and yogurt, sprinkles some black pepper over the mixture. The salad should be split evenly between the two pieces of bread. Dish up.

134.   Watermelon Salsa with Grilled Grouper

What we need:

- 4 grouper fillets, skin on, measuring 4 ounces each
- ¼ tsp. of freshly grated black pepper
- 2 cups of watermelon that has been coarsely diced and is seedless
- ¼ cup of red onion that has been coarsely chopped
- 1 Serrano pepper, de-veined, deseeded, and cut very finely
- 1 medium-sized clove of garlic, minced
- 1 ½ tsp. of fresh cilantro, coarsely chopped, and set aside.
- 1 milliliter of lime juice that has been freshly squeezed

Cooking Method:

1. Take the bowl provided and combine all of the elements for the salsa. Put it in the refrigerator for a while to chill.

2. Place your grill cooker over a high-medium flame and sprinkle it with oil to grease it.

3. Add some grated black pepper to the grouper. Cook the grouper with the skin facing down for 5 to 7 minutes.

4. Cook the grouper, tossing it often, for another six minutes over medium heat, until it is browned and easily flakes apart.

5. Take the fish off the grill and serve it right away with the watermelon salsa.

135. Waffle Sandwich

What we need:

- 1 (1.33-ounce) solidified multigrain waffle
- 2 tbsp. cream cheese, mollified
- 2 tsp. dark-colored sugar
- Ground cinnamon (¼ tsp.)
- 1 tbsp. of raisins
- 1 tbsp. hacked pecans, toasted

Cooking Method:

1. Toast waffles as per bundle headings.

2. Blend cream cheese, dark sugar, and cinnamon until very well mixed. Spread the cream cheese blend over the waffles. Sprinkle with raisins and pecans.

3. Cut the waffle down the middle. Sandwich waffle parts together with filling inside.

136. Bagel sandwich

What we need:

- ½ cup (4 ounces) goat cheddar, disintegrated
- 4 ounces cheese cream mollified
- 1 tbsp. of honey
- 1/3 cup hacked toasted pecans
- 1 cinnamon-raisin twirl small bagel, split and toasted
- ¼ cup red Anjou pear, unpeeled and meagerly cut

Cooking Method:

1. Consolidate the initial three ingredients in a little bowl. Mix in pecans.

2. Spread 1 tbsp. of goat cheddar uniformly onto the cut sides of the bagel.

3. Spot pear cuts on the base portion of the bagel. Supplant the bagel top.

4. Spread and chill, staying spread for as long as a week.

137.   Almond-cranberry cereal bar

What we need:

- Almond margarine (½ cup)

- Sugar (2/3 cup)

- 5 cups of fresh wheat grain squares

- Dried cranberries (3/4 cup)

- ½ cup fragmented almonds, toasted

- Cooking shower

Cooking Method:

1. Spoon almond margarine and honey into a large Dutch broiler. Boil on medium heat. Blend with oats, cranberries, and almonds, hurling to coat.

2. Put the blend into a prepared dish covered with a cooking splash, squeezing it into an even layer with cling wrap.

3. Let stand 1 hour so that sets. Cut it into 12 bars.

138.   Chewy Date-Apple Bars

What we need:

- Two and a half cups for the entire set of dates

- 1 cup of dried apples

- ½ cup pecans, toasted

- ½ cup rolled oats

- ¼ tsp. ground cinnamon

Cooking Method:

1. Bring the oven down to 350 degrees.

2. Put the initial three ingredients into a blender and mix until the leafy foods are finely slashed.

3. Include oats and cinnamon; beat 8 to multiple times so that soggy and oats are cleaved. Blend into a delicately lubed 9 x 5-inch portion container, squeezing into an even layer with a saran cover.

4. Heat for 15 minutes at 350°F. Cool completely in a dish on a line rack. Then cut into 12 bars.

139. Cherry Scones

What we need:

- 9 ounces of flour (around 2 cups)
- Salt
- Sugar (¼ cup)
- Heating powder (one and a half tsp.)
- ¼ cup chilled, unsalted margarine
- 3/4 cup dried tart fruits, slashed
- Fat-free buttermilk (3/4 cup)
- Cooking shower
- 1 tbsp. turbaned sugar (discretionary)

Cooking Method:

1. Bring the oven down to 425°.

2. Estimate or softly spoon flour into dry measuring cups; then, smooth with a blade.

3. Consolidate the salt, powder, flour, and sugar in a big dish, combining admirably with a whisker. Then cut in the spread, utilizing a good blender, until the blend looks like coarse supper. Blend in fruits.

4. Include buttermilk and almonds separately whenever wanted, mixing just until damp.

5. Mix the butter onto a daintily floured exterior and massage lightly multiple times, including with floured hands. Structure the mixture in an 8-inch saucepan on a prepared sheet covered with parchment paper.

6. Cut the butter into 10 wedges, slicing into but not through the combination. Coat the top of the butter with cooking spray. Sprinkle with turbinate sugar whenever desired.

7. Keep the preparation sheet on a rack on the stove. Heat it at 425° for 20 minutes, so that is brilliant.

140. Zucchini Chicken Thighs

What we need:

- 1 cup of raw quinoa
- 1 cubic millimeter of extra-virgin olive oil
- Chicken flesh
- ½ jar (6 oz) of quartered marinated crab hearts, drained
- ½ tbsp. freshly squeezed lemon juice
- I cut one medium-sized zucchini into small pieces.

Cooking Method:

1. Cook the quinoa in accordance with the directions provided on the box.
2. Heat oil in a large pan over high heat until just before boiling. Maintain this temperature until usage.
3. If you want the chicken to have a golden brown color, roast it for two minutes on each side.
4. Continue to simmer for another five to ten minutes, ensuring that both the chicken and the zucchini are well cooked.
5. After adding the crab hearts and bringing the whole liquid back up to a boil, keep cooking it for a few minutes more. Take the pan off the heat, and after its cool enough to handle, drizzle some lemon juice over the top of it.
6. Accompany the dish with quinoa.

141. Balsamic Baked Fish with Broccoli

Ingredients

- Chop two broccoli heads into smaller pieces. ¼ tsp. of dried thyme
- ¼ tsp. of dried onion flakes
- Olive oil 2 tbsp.
- ¾ a cup of vinegar, each split
- Lemon sap 1 tbsp.
- Black pepper to taste
- Spray for cooking that doesn't stick

Cooking Method:

1. Bring the oven's temperature up to 450 degrees Fahrenheit.

2. Add thyme leaves, black pepper, and onion powder to the fish, and then stir it to fry.

3. Coat the baking surface with oil sprits, and then arrange the salmon fillets on the sheet.

4. Place the broccoli stalks in a circle around them, and then drizzle one tbsp. of olive oil over them all.

5. After adding peppers to the dish, put it in the oven and let it cook for 15 minutes.

6. In the meantime, combine the remaining olive oil, balsamic vinegar, and lemon juice in a saucepan set over medium heat and stir until well combined. Maintain a low boil for the mixture for five minutes, after which it has reached the desired consistency.

7. After baking, sprinkle vinegar sauce on the fish before serving.

142. Chickpea Veggie Sauté

What we need:

- ½ of a can of chickpeas with reduced sodium, which has been drained and washed.

- 7 cans of low-sodium chopped tomatoes, each weighing 7 ounces

- 2 cloves of garlic, diced up

- 2 cups of spinach for infants

- 1 tbsp. of olive oil, extra-virgin

- ½ tsp. of curry powder

- 1 eighth of a tsp. of new black pepper

Cooking Method:

1. Over a medium heat setting, bring the oil to the desired temperature in a cooker. Garlic should be cooked for thirty seconds, or until it takes on a soft consistency.

2. Cook the chickpeas, tomatoes, and curry powder in the saucepan until they are cooked. Pepper should be used as the seasoning.

3. Bring the mixture to a boil and continue to cook it for the subsequent half an hour, making sure to stir it more often.

4. Following the addition of the spinach, let it continue to be tossed for the subsequent two minutes until it has wilted And to be of assistance.

143. Cod Parcels with Mushrooms and Spinach

What we need:

- 4 cups of baby spinach
- A measure and a half of sliced shiitake mushrooms
- 4 fish fillets, 4 ounces each
- Old Bay seasoning, ½ of a tsp.
- Grated black pepper 1 tsp.
- Add a cup of chopped scallions, including both the green and white portions.
- Olive oil 2 tbsp.

Cooking Method:

1. Bring the oven's temperature to 425 degrees Fahrenheit. Rupture four square pieces of aluminum foil that measure twelve inches each. Each piece of foil should contain one cup of greens and one-half cup of mushrooms.

2. Put one piece of fish on top of the vegetables and season it with pepper and Old Bay. Scatter the sliced scallions over the top, and then sprinkle with the oil.

3. Seal and encapsulate cod by folding packets into airtight packaging. Bake the packets for 15 minutes on parchment paper. Remove the casserole from the oven. Carefully unfold the sachets.

144. Grilled Garlic-Lime Chicken

What we need:

- Skinless chicken breasts weighing a total of one pound
- 2 tbsp. of olive oil
- A single lime's worth of grated rind and juice
- 2 garlic cloves cut very coarsely
- Use freshly grated black pepper for seasoning.

Cooking Method:

1. Prepare the grill by heating it to a temperature between medium and high.

2. Place the meat pieces in one coat on an ovenproof plate, and then place the dish in the oven. Individual taste should determine the amount of oil, lime juice, lime zest, garlic, and black pepper to add.

3. Give it a thorough toss to guarantee even coating, and then marinate it for the next 10 minutes.

4. To begin, spray the rack of your barbecue with oil. Next, combine the chicken with the other ingredients and cook it for four to five minutes on each side. Help out with.

145. Salmon with Pomegranate Salsa

What we need:

- Breasts of skinless chicken weighing in at a total of one pound
- 2 tbsp. of olive oil
- Lime rind and juice were added.
- Two salmon fillets
- 2 tsp. grated black pepper
- 1 segment of lemon
- A little less than half a cup's worth of pomegranate seeds
- ¼ of a cube of cucumber, chopped
- ⅛ of a tsp. of red onion, minced
- 1 tsp. of fresh dill that has been chopped
- Lemon juice is equal to one-fourth of a fruit's volume.

Cooking Method:

1. Place a baking sheet inside the oven and begin preheating by raising the temperature to 450°F.
2. Spread out the salmon fillets on a baking sheet in a single layer, and then cover the fish with oil. Bake for fifteen minutes. Serve lemon slices on the side and sprinkle with black pepper.
3. Place the steak in the oven and roast it for approximately 15 minutes, or until it resembles flaky fish in texture.
4. While you wait, use the medium bowl at your disposal to combine the pomegranate seeds, cucumber, onion, dill, the remaining salt, and the lemon juice.
5. Just before serving, arrange the salsa in an attractive pattern on top of the salmon.

146. Pumpkin Cakes

What we need:

- ¼ cup of pumpkin puree
- 1 tsp. of almond milk, unsweetened
- 4 tsp. pure honey
- 2 tbsp. of olive oil
- 1 tsp. of baking powder
- ¼ cup of oat flour
- A pinch of salt

Cooking Method:

1. Position a baking tray inside the preheated oven and turn the temperature up to 350 degrees.

2. Combine the almond butter, pumpkin purée, and pumpkin pie spice in a small measuring dish. Honey, milk, olive oil, and the spice of pumpkin pie are the ingredients in this recipe.

3. Combine all of the dry components (salt, flour, and baking powder) in a basin designated for mixing.

4. Muffins are done when a toothpick inserted in the middle shows no residue after 22-25 minutes in a preheated oven.

5. The mixture should be distributed in an even layer between two ramekins that are each 4 ounces in capacity.

6. Sprinkle an additional amount of the pumpkin pie spice over each serving.

147. Marinated Berries

Cooking Method:

- 1 cup of blueberries, if you want them
- 2 cups of fresh strawberries, cutted
- 1 tbsp. of natural honey
- 1/8 of a tsp. of new black pepper
- A tbsp worth of balsamic vinegar
- 2 tbsp. of mint, finely chopped

Cooking Method:

1. Combine the strawberries, blueberries (if desired), honey, and cinnamon in a large bowl.

2. Combine the pepper, mint (if using it), and vinegar in a big basin that is not reactive.

3. Give the flavors some time to come together for no less than 25 minutes and up to 2 hours.

148. Carrot Cookies with Chocolate Chip

Cooking Method:

- 1 egg, big in size
- A third of a cup of almond meal
- A quarter cup of shredded carrots
- ⅛ cup of applesauce that has not been sweetened
- A quarter of a cup of dairy-free dark-colored chocolate chips
- 1 milliliter of unadulterated maple syrup
- ¼ tsp. of the baking powder
- ½ tsp. of cinnamon powder

Cooking Method:

1. Turn up the microwave. Prepare a parchment paper lining for your baking sheet.

2. In an enormous combining bowl, whisk the almond nutrition, baking powder, chocolate chips, carrots, applesauce, maple syrup, eggs, as well as grated cinnamon. Combine all of the ingredients by stirring each other until the mixture takes on the texture of thick dough.

3. Place tbsp.-sized rounds onto the baking sheet that has been prepared. Bake the bread for ten to fifteen minutes, so that it begins to become a light brown color. Dish up.

149. Roasted Peas

What we need:

- 1 can (15 ounces) of peas, emptied and flushed
- 1 tbsp. olive oil
- 1 tsp. ground cumin
- ½ tsp. smoked paprika
- 1 tsp. of garlic paste
- 1 tsp. sea salt

Cooking Method:

1. When peas fall into a colander, keep their silky, light surface.

2. For crunch, gently wipe peas dry with a clean dish towel or piece towel.

3. On a parchment-lined baking pan, dried peas make mild beans light and crisp. Think about how much oil will crisp each pea, and taste it. Add floor cumin, smoked paprika, garlic powder, and sea salt to the peas for flavor.

4. For an even taste, gently arrange the peas on the baking sheet and coat each bean with oil and spice mix.

5. Burn peas evenly until brittle in an unmarried layer. To produce crispy peas, place the baking sheet in the oven.

6. Visualize the humorous metamorphosis by toasting the peas for 28–32 minutes until golden and crispy.

7. Check the peas on a regular basis, and gently bounce the baking sheet to promote even browning and a lovely kitchen smell. Peas are crisp when chilled, so let them cool before eating.

150. Turkey Burgers

What we need:

- 4 grouper fillets, skin on, measuring 4 ounces each
- ¼ tsp. of freshly grated black pepper
- **With regard to the salsa:**
- Chop two cups of watermelon coarsely and ensure it is seedless.
- ¼ cup of red onion that has been coarsely chopped
- 1 Serrano pepper, de-veined, deseeded, and cut very finely
- 1 medium-sized clove of garlic, minced
- 1 ½ tsp. of fresh cilantro, coarsely chopped, and set aside.
- Use one milliliter of freshly squeezed lime juice.

Cooking Method:

1. Mix the salsa items in the small dish provided. Put it in the refrigerator for a while to chill.
2. Spread some oil over your grill pan and set it over medium heat.
3. Add some grated black pepper to the grouper. Cook the grouper with the skin facing down for 5 to 7 minutes.
4. Cook the grouper for another 6 minutes on medium heat, turning it regularly, until it is brown and readily flakes apart.
5. Take the fish off the grill and serve it right away with the watermelon salsa.

151. Roasted mixed nuts

What we need:

- 1 ounce of raw, assorted nuts
- 1 egg white
- ½ tsp. of water
- ½ tsp. of cumin powder
- ¼ tsp. of sea salt
- ⅛ tsp of garlic powder
- The appropriate amount of grated cayenne pepper

Cooking Method:

1. In order to get the oven ready, put a cookie sheet inside of it, and then turn the temperature up to 300 degrees Fahrenheit. To prepare a baking sheet, first spray it with cooking spray and then line it with parchment paper.

2. Egg whites and water should be combined and whisked together in a basin of about medium size until the mixture begins to froth.

3. Coat the nuts by mixing them around in the basin. Place a strainer with a fine mesh over the sink, and pour the coated nuts into it. Toss the nuts to eliminate any extra water. Put it to the side.

4. Mix the cumin, salt, cayenne pepper, and garlic powder in a big bag that can be sealed back up.

5. Lay the nuts in the paper bag, then seal it and wobble it vigorously to fully cover the nuts with the spice mixture.

6. On the baking sheet, spread the nuts out in a single layer and roast them for approximately 20 minutes, or until they are golden and dry.

7. Allow the nuts to fully cool while they are still on the baking pan. Dish up.

152. Baked Tortilla Chips

What we need:

- Olive oil, one tbsp.

- 4 medium-sized tortillas made from whole wheat

- ¼ tsp. of salt

Cooking Method:

1. Increase the degree of heat in the oven to 355 degrees Fahrenheit. Oil the inside and outside of each tortilla using the brush dipped in oil.

2. Place the tortilla pieces in one layer on a baking tray with a rim. A pinch of salt should be sprinkled on top of each chip.

3. 3. Put them in the oven for exactly ten minutes, then turn them over and put them back in the oven for exactly three to five minutes more until they are golden brown. Dish up.

153. Veggie Burger

What we need:

- 2 tbsp. of olive oil
- 4 big Portobello mushrooms, cleaned and trimmed of their stems and gills
- 1 tbsp. of minced garlic
- 4 crusty rolls made with healthy grains
- ½ cups of goat cheese in crushed form
- Black pepper that has been freshly grated, to taste (optional)
- 4 lettuce leaves, green in color

Cooking Method:

1. Set the oven's temperature to four hundred twenty-five degrees Fahrenheit. Aluminum foil should be used to line the rimmed baking sheet you have.
2. In a separate, smaller dish, mix the garlic and oil together. After applying roughly half of the mixture with a brush to both surfaces of the mushrooms, let them sit aside for ten minutes to marinate.
3. In the meantime, cut the rolls in half lengthwise. On the opposite side of each roll, brush some of the garlic oil that was left over.
4. Distribute about 2 tsp. of goat cheese on top of each roll.
5. Arrange the mushrooms in a layer on parchment paper and roast them in the microwave for ten minutes on both sides.
6. On the underside of every roll, set a single mushroom. If you like it spicy, add some pepper. After that, place the top of the roll on top of a cabbage leaf.

154. Roasted Masala Chickpeas

What we need:

- A tsp. of cumin powder
- Cooked chickpeas, dried, and skin removed
- A tsp. of asafoetida (hing)
- Ghee or coconut oil
- Ground paprika 1 tsp.
- A pinch of coriander powder
- A tsp. of ground black salt

Cooking method:

1. In a bowl, combine the chickpeas that have been dried with the ghee or coconut oil that has been melted.

2. In a mixing bowl, combine some ground asafoetida, black salt, black pepper, cumin powder, coriander powder, and ground paprika.

3. Spread the chickpeas out in a single layer on a baking sheet and roast them in the oven at 400 degrees for 20 to 25 minutes to get a crispy texture.

4. After allowing them to cool, dig into these Ayurvedic Roasted Masala Chickpeas for a satisfying snack that's also high in protein.

155. Berry and Nut Mix

What we need:

- Mixed nuts (e.g., almonds, cashews, and walnuts)
- Mixed dried berries
- A tsp. of ground cinnamon
- Shredded coconut
- A tsp. of crushed nutmeg
- A tsp. of crushed cloves
- A tsp. of grated cardamom

Cooking method:

1. Mix together in a bowl the assorted dried berries, the assorted nuts, the shredded coconut, and the powdered cinnamon, the grated cardamom, the crushed cloves, and the crushed nutmeg.

2. Combine thoroughly.

3. Enjoy this Ayurvedic Berry and Nut Mix as a sweet and crunchy snack.

156. Toasted Sweet Potato Fries

What we need:

- 2 big sweet potatoes, sliced into French fry-sized pieces
- Olive oil 2 tbsp.
- Garlic powder 1 tsp.
- ¼ tsp. of salt

- A very small amount of grated cayenne pepper

Cooking Method:

1. Setting the oven to 425°F is the first step. Use parchment paper on your baking sheet.

2. Mix sweet potatoes, garlic powder, oil, salt, and cayenne pepper in a large basin.

3. Arrange them on the baking sheet so that they form a single layer.

4. Toast sweet potatoes on a roasting sheet for 35-40 minutes to achieve desired crispiness.

5. Take the dish out of the oven, and then serve.

157. Mixed Vegetable Chips

What we need:

- Olive oil cooking spray

- 2 medium beets, skinned and chopped

- 1 medium zucchini, chopped

- 1 medium sweet potato, chopped

- 1 small rutabaga, peeled and sliced

- ¼ tsp salt

- ¼ tsp. dried rosemary

Cooking Method:

1. Put the oven on for preheating. Cooking spray should be sprayed onto a baking sheet.

2. On the baking sheet that has been prepared in advance, spread the vegetables out in a single layer, and then spray them with cooking spray. Roast the veggies until they reach the desired consistency.

3. Put it in the heated oven and bake for about half an hour to an hour, or until the top is browned.

4. After 10 minutes, give the veggies a flip and continue to cook until they are crisp. Remove it from the oven and put aside. Place the food on a paper-towel-lined dish to drain excess oil.

5. Combine the salt and the rosemary in the smaller bowl you have. Add some rosemary salt to the chips and season them lightly.

158.   Cakes Made With Polenta

What we need:

- 1 cup of cornmeal, finely grated
- 5 cups of water
- Garlic powder ½ tsp.
- ¼ tsp. of salt
- Spray for cooking with olive oil.
- 2 tbsp. of olive oil

Cooking Method:

1. You will need to use high heat in order to bring the water in the large pot you have been using up to a boil.

2. While steadily whisking, start adding the cornmeal to the water in little increments. You will need to use high heat in order to bring the water in the large pot you have been using to a boil.

3. Keep boiling the cornmeal with the heat turned down until it is entirely cooked, which should take anywhere between 25 and 30 minutes, turning it often, or until it has thickened. Take it away from the heat immediately.

4. While you wait, prepare a baking dish measuring 9 by ½ inches by spraying it with oil spray and lining it with baking parchment.

5. Place the batter in the baking dish that has been prepared and chill it in the fridge for at least an hour, or until it has reached the desired consistency.

6. Slice the polenta into twelve pieces, or, if you prefer, use a circular cookie cutter to form cakes out of the polenta.

7. Bring the oil to a temperature of medium-high in the big skillet you have.

8. After the polenta cakes have been mixed, they should be browned on the outside by cooking them for around two to three minutes more per side. After taking the cooker off the flame, the meal may then be served.

159. Edamame with Sesame and Garlic

What we need:

- 1 container of frozen edamame with its shells intact
- Olive oil, one tbsp.
- A tbsp. and a half of toasted olive oil
- Garlic cloves 4
- ½ milliliter of kosher salt
- ¼ tsp. or more of dried red pepper flakes

Cooking Method:

1. Over high heat, bring the water contained in the large saucepan to a boil. After adding the edamame, continue to simmer for another two to three minutes, or until it is completely warm.

2. Additionally, in the large skillet that you have been using, heat the salt, olive oil, garlic, sesame oil, and crushed red chili flakes in the skillet for one to two minutes over medium heat; after that, take the pan away from the burner.

3. After draining the edamame, put it in the pan and toss it so that everything is combined. Dish up.

160. Crispy Potato

What we need:

- Dried rosemary 1 tsp.
- 2 russet potatoes
- Olive oil frying spray
- Pepper and salt to taste
- 1/8 of a tsp. of new pepper

Cooking Method:

1. Preheat the oven to 375 degrees F by turning the temperature dial.

2. Arrange potatoes in a dish that can be heated in the microwave, and cook them for five minutes at high power.

3. Turn the potatoes over and continue cooking them in the microwave for another three to four minutes, or until they are soft.

4. Crack the potatoes in half and take away the meat with a spoon.

5. Coat the outside of each potato with oil spray, and then spice it with rosemary and black pepper.

6. Put them on the baking pan and bake them for anywhere from 5 to 10 minutes, or until they are crispy. Dish up.

161.   Rosemary-Roasted Almonds

What we need:

- 2 cups of raw almonds, unsalted and in their natural state
- 1 ½ tbsp. of olive oil
- 2 ¼ tsp. of freshly chopped rosemary

Cooking Method:

1. To preheat the oven, adjust the thermostat dial to 350 degrees F.

2. Put all of the items, such as the almonds, into the bowl, and thoroughly combine them all together so that the almonds are evenly coated.

3. Place the mixture on a baking sheet and bake it at a temperature of 400 degrees Fahrenheit for duration of 10-15 minutes, stirring it twice, until it reaches a golden brown color. To be served.

162.   Crispy kale snacks

What we need:

- 1 bunch of curly kale
- 2 tsp. of olive oil
- ⅛ Tsp. of kosher salt

Cooking Method:

1. To begin, turn on the oven so that it may begin to heat up. In order to get a baking sheet ready for use, you must first line it with parchment paper and then give it a rim.

2. Remove the rough stems from the kale and break the leaves into squares approximately the size of large potato chips (the squares will become smaller after the kale has been cooked).

3. After spraying the kale with oil and placing it in a big dish, tear the kale into bite-sized pieces using your fingers. Massage the kale for one to two minutes to ensure that it is evenly coated. Distribute evenly on the sheet of baking parchment.

4. Cook for eight minutes, give them a stir, and then continue cooking for another seven minutes before checking on them.

5. Remove them from the oven promptly as they have a crisp texture, which should be within the next five minutes. After salting, the dish is ready to be served.

163.   Spiced Popcorn with Ghee

What we need:

- Ground black salt 1 tsp.
- Popped popcorn
- A tsp. of asafoetida (hing)
- Ghee (clarified butter)
- Turmeric powder 1 tsp.
- A bit of black pepper

Cooking method:

1. In a large bowl, sprinkle hot, popped popcorn with melted ghee.
2. Sprinkle with turmeric powder, ground black salt, black pepper, and asafoetida.
3. To achieve a uniform coating on the popcorn, give it a good toss.
4. This Spiced Popcorn with Ghee makes for a delicious and savory snack that you may enjoy.

164.   Asparagus Fries

What we need:

- ½ bunch of asparagus, with the tough ends taken off and the stalks split lengthwise.
- 1 egg that has been beaten
- 1 tsp. of grated mustard
- ¼ cup of bread crumbs
- ½ tsp. of dried garlic
- ⅛ Tsp. of salt

Cooking Method:

1. Prepare the oven for cooking at 400°F by turning it on. In order to get your baking sheet ready, you need to line it with a sheet of parchment.

2. Get a bowl and put the beaten egg in it. Put everything else, save the asparagus, into a separate dish and mix well.

3. The next step is to dip each length of asparagus in the egg that has been beaten, and then proceed to coat it with the breadcrumb mixture. After that, arrange the coated asparagus on the roasting sheet that has been prepared, taking care not to crowd the asparagus too much.

4. Make sure the topping is crispy in the oven, which should take no more than 15 minutes. Serve.

165.   Apple Slices with Nut Butter

What we need:

- Crisp and juicy sliced apples for a refreshing and naturally sweet base
- Nut butter for a light and nutty space
- Optional toppings:
- Honey, for a touch of sweetness
- Chia seeds provide additional surface area and nutrients.
- For a warm and aromatic taste, use cinnamon.
- Slivered almonds or other nuts for a delightful crunch

Cooking Method:

1. Clean and slice the apple into thin, manageable slices, expecting each piece's crispness and natural sweetness.

2. Place the apple pieces on a plate, hoping for a colorful and attractive presentation.

3. Spoon a significant amount of your best nut butter onto each apple slice, distributing it evenly with the back of the spoon, hoping for a light and kind layer.

4. If desired, sprinkle a tiny amount of honey over the nut butter, guessing the subtle sweetness and improving the flavors.

5. Sprinkle chia seeds on top of the nut butter, guessing the counted texture and nutritional benefits they provide.

6. Lightly sprinkle cinnamon over the apple slices, expecting the warm and comforting aroma to infuse the snack.

7. Sprinkle sliced almonds or nuts over the apple pieces, envisioning the satisfying crunch and extra-nutty flavor.

8. Serve the apple slices with nut butter instantly, savoring the combination of crisp apple, creamy nut butter, and optional toppings.

166. Avocado and Tuna Salad Sandwich

What we need:

- 1 water-packed can of tuna weighing five ounces, drained
- 1 ripe avocado with the pit removed, the peel removed, and the flesh sliced 2 scallions, both the green and white sections minced
- ½ lemon juice
- 2 tbsp. of olive oil
- Pepper, black, freshly grated, one-fourth of a tsp.
- 4 pieces of bread made with whole wheat

Cooking Method:

1. Put everything except the breads in the smaller bowl and stir to combine.
2. 2. Distribute the tuna filling over two pieces of bread using a spatula. Assemble the sandwich, and then serve it.

167. Homemade Popcorn

What we need:

- Popcorn kernels are the foundation of fluffy and crispy popcorn.
- Cooking oil for popping the kernels
- For a rich and buttery flavor (optional), melt butter.
- Salt, to taste, for seasoning (optional)

Optional toppings:

- Grated Parmesan cheese for a savory and cheesy twist
- Caramel sauce for a sweet and indulgent treat
- For a spicy kick, add chili powder.
- Dried herbs (such as rosemary or thyme) for a fragrant and herbaceous touch

Cooking Method:

1. A saucepan or stovetop popcorn popper will pop popcorn over low-to-medium heat.
2. As you oil the pot base, imagine the kernels sizzling. Put a few popcorn seeds in the saucepan and cover it until they pop to signal the oil is ready.

3. After the test kernels pop, take them from the cooker and count the popcorn, envisioning the excitement. To release steam without retaining kernels, cover the pot with a little ajar.

4. While gently shaking the pot over heat, imagine the kernels dancing and creating fluffy popcorn. Hop the pot until most kernels pop and the sound slows. Before gently removing the cooker from heat with the lid on, any leftover kernels should pop.

5. Take off the lid and imagine a popcorn cloud. Pour it on, and imagine each popcorn kernel covered in buttery goodness.

6. Add salt to taste for the correct herb balance on popcorn. For flavor, sprinkle popcorn with grated Parmesan cheese, caramel spice, chili powder, or dry herbs.

7. If the flavors are different, gently toss the popcorn to distribute the toppings.

8. Handmade popcorn in large bowls or individual serving dishes is delightful.

168. Whole Grain Crackers with Tuna Salad

What we need:

- For a nutritious and crunchy base, 1 box of whole grain crackers
- 2 cans of canned tuna in water, drained and flaked, for a protein-packed salad
- Mayonnaise, ½ cup, for creaminess and flavor
- Dijon mustard, 1 tbsp., for a tangy kick
- Red onion, ¼ cup, finely chopped, for a mild onion flavor and added crunch
- Celery, ¼ cup, finely chopped
- Pickles or pickle relish, 2 tbsp.
- Lemon juice 1 tbsp.
- Pepper and salt, to taste, for seasoning

Cooking Method:

1. Mix flaked tuna, mayonnaise, Dijon mustard, sliced red onion, celery, pickles or jam relish, lemon juice, salt, and pepper in a dish to make a wonderful tuna salad.

2. Mix the ingredients carefully to coat the tuna with the light dressing, and distribute the flavors throughout the salad. Adjust the tuna salad seasoning with salt, pepper, or lemon juice to taste.

3. If desired, carefully add chopped fresh herbs, cherry tomatoes, or avocado to the salad, envisioning its brilliant colors and freshness. Cover the dish with a flexible cloth and refrigerate the tuna salad for 30 minutes to cool the flavors.

4. Place whole-grain crackers on a tray or plate to serve, anticipating their freshness and healthiness. Spread a generous quantity of cold tuna salad on each cracker, and imagine the range of textures and flavors.

5. Garnish with fresh herbs for visual appeal. Expect protein, whole seeds, and fresh ingredients in each mouthful of Whole

6. Grain crackers with tuna salad are a tasty and healthy snack or light entrée. Store leftover tuna salad in the fridge for three **Day** s; use it as a snack or sandwich.

DRINKS

169.   Banana-Avocado Smoothie

What we need:

- ½ a pitted avocado
- 1 peeled banana
- 1 tbsp. of honey
- Fat-free milk

Cooking Method:

1. To begin, place all of the components into the food processor, and then run the machine until the mixture is totally smooth.

2. Serve it in a glass, and you can mix ice cubes if you want.

170.   Chia Peach Smoothies

What we need:

- 1 peach, cut into quarters, and pitted.
- 1 fluid ounce of almond milk, unsweetened
- ¼ tsp. of honey
- A tbsp.ful of rolled oats
- A quarter of a tsp. of grated ginger, grated nutmeg, and grated cloves
- ⅛ tsp. of grated cinnamon in addition to cardamom powder
- 2 pieces of ice

Cooking Method:

1. Put everything into a blender and blitz until it forms a smooth mixture.

2. Serve at once as part of the morning meal.

171. Berry Breakfast

What we need:

- ¾ Almond milk
- 1 icy catcall
- 2 tsp. revived orange juice
- ¼ freezing cherries
- Honey to test
- 1 tsp. bottom flaxseed

Cooking Method:

1. Mix all elements in a blender, counting lemon sap to taste.
2. Stir until smooth. Flow into two relaxed drinks.

172. Best Smoothie

What we need:

- 1 banana
- Simple, nonfat curd
- 1 orange juice
- 7 frozen strawberries

Cooking Method:

1. Mix the juice, banana, strawberries, and curd for 25 seconds.
2. Rub down the flanks and mix for an extra 10 seconds.

173. Pineapple Filling

What we need:

- 6 ices
- 1 c. low-fat curd
- 1 c. pineapple chunks

Cooking Method:

1. Mix the curd and ice cubes and mix in a blender, added if you want, until the ice is crushed into small pieces.

2. Mix the pineapple, and then blend until smooth.

174. Strawberry Smoothie

What we need:

- 1½ tsp. honey
- Milk
- 1 ripe banana,
- Chopped 7 fresh strawberries

Cooking Method:

1. Mix the milk, strawberries, banana, and honey.

2. Decant until it gets smooth.

175. Papaya Perfection

What we need:

- 1 cup of normal curd
- 1 papaya, chopped into cubes
- ½ ice cubes
- ½ tsp. coconut essence
- ½ fresh pineapple cubes
- 1 tsp. of linseed

Cooking Method:

1. Blend the curd, papaya, ice, pineapple, coconut essence, and linseed.

2. Blend for approximately 40 seconds.

176. Peachy Smoothie

What we need:

- ½ cup diced strawberries
- 1 cup of milk
- ½ cup frozen peaches

- 3 crushed ice cubes
- 2 tbsp. of curd
- 2 tsp. of whey protein powder

Cooking Method:

1. Blend all elements with liquids like curd, milk, and juice. This will assist in cracking down and making sure it's nicely spread.

2. Blend all elements, like oatmeal and fruit, and then mix ice at the end.

3. You can chuck additional ice cubes for a more comprehensive shake, counting volume about the calories.

177. Mango Apricot

What we need:

- 3 ripe mangoes,
- 1 plain or low-fat curd
- 8 ice cubes and lemon peel to decorate
- 7 apricots diced
- 4 tsp. of fresh lemon pulp

Cooking Method:

1. Blend all the elements in a blender. Blend it for 20 seconds. Mix the ice cubes and blend for 9 to 10 seconds, until it gets thick or smooth.

2. Flow into glasses, decorate with lemon peel if you want, and enjoy.

178. Watermelon Smoothie

What we need:

- Milk
- Crushed ice
- 3 cups chopped watermelon

Cooking Method:

1. Blend all elements for 25 seconds, until it gets thick or smooth.

2. Mix the ice and blend for another 25 seconds, or to your preferred thickness.

179. Berry Smoothie

What we need:

- 2 Blueberries
- 2 diced strawberries
- 3 tbsp. of honey
- 2 Raspberries
- Ice cubes
- ½ tsp. fresh lemon sap

Cooking Method:

1. Mix all the elements in a juicer and blend.
2. Blend it until it is completely creamy.

180. Sunrise Smoothie

What we need:

- 1 cup frozen and chopped apricot
- 1 ripe banana
- 1 container of curd
- 1 tbsp. chilled lemonade
- ½ cup cold soda

Cooking Method:

1. Place all of the components in a blender and mix them. Blend it until it is completely creamy.
2. Mix in the cold soda as much as you want and enjoy.

181. Exceptional Berry Smoothie

What we need:

- 1 cup of diced and frozen strawberries
- ½ cup cold lemon sap
- 1 cup diced and frozen berries

Cooking Method:

1. Mix the lemon sap, raspberries, and strawberries, then blend.

2. Mix until it becomes slippery.

182. Fruity Smoothie

What we need:

- 1 cup crushed pineapple
- 1 cup of frozen strawberries
- ½ cup normal curd

Cooking Method:

1. Mix the curd and frozen strawberries in a mixer for 50 seconds.

2. Make a drink and mix a spoonful of linseed oil, then drink with a spoonful of pumpkin or sunflower seeds.

183. Dieting Smoothie

What we need:

- 1 cup of curd
- 1 cup of orange sap
- 2 cups chilled blueberries, like any berries, strawberries, or raspberries

Cooking Method:

1. Place the berries, orange sap, and curd in a mixer and beat for 40 seconds.

2. Mix for 40 seconds, or as soon as it gets smooth.

184. Soy Smoothie

What we need:

- 1 chilled banana cut into small slices
- 1 cup chilled berries
- 2 cups cornflakes
- 2 cups of any flavor of soy milk

Cooking Method:

1. Blend the cornflakes, banana, and blueberries with soy milk in a mixer for 40 seconds.

2. Rub the flanks and combine for an extra 30 seconds.

185.   Madness of Mango

What we need:

- Crushed ice
- 2 cup pineapple pieces
- 1 ripe banana, diced
- 1 cup ripe, chopped mango
- 2 cups chilled, any flavor curd

Cooking Method:

1. Blend the pineapple, chilled curd, mango, and banana. Coordinate until smoothie.
2. Slowly sink sufficient ice into the running blender to get the rank up to 3 cups. Mix until the combined gravy and ice are maximally crushed and mixed well with juice.

186.   Oat Smoothie

What we need:

- 1 cup of oats
- 1 sliced banana
- 1 tsp.   maple sap
- 2 cup chopped strawberries
- of almonds 1 cup
- 1 cup of curd

Cooking Method:

1. Get all the elements together, and then mix them in the blender.
2. Serve

187.   Curd-Mango Smoothie

What we need:

- 2 tbsp. of honey
- 1 cup chilled mango, chopped
- 1 cup of curd
- 1 tsp.   cinnamon

Cooking Method:

1. Get all the elements together, and then mix them in the blender.

2. Serve

188.   Parsley Salad Smoothie

- 1 cup of any kind of parsley or green leaf salad that you desire
- 1 cup almonds, chopped
- 2 cups grated cucumbers
- 1 cup of coconut milk

Cooking Method:

1. Get all the elements together, and then mix them in the blender.

2. Serve.

189.   Saffron and cashew milk

What we need:

- Crushed cashews for garnish
- 1 glass of Cashew milk (or any preferred milk)
- A pinch of Saffron threads
- 1 tsp. of Ghee or coconut oil
- 2 tsp. of Honey

Cooking method:

1. It is recommended that the cashew milk be warmed in a saucepan set over low heat.

2. After the saffron threads have been added, the milk needs some time to fully absorb its flavor before it can be served.

3. To sweeten, either honey may be used.

4. The cashews should be broken up into smaller pieces before being used as a garnish for the warm meal.

5. This Ayurvedic Saffron and Cashew Milk is the ideal beverage to serve with your sweet course because of its luxurious texture and heady aroma.

190.   Cardamom and Date Smoothies

What we need:

- 2 Chopped dates for garnish
- 1 tsp. of Cardamom powder
- 2 Dates, pitted
- 1 glass of Almond milk
- 1 tbsp. of Yogurt or dairy-free yogurt

Cooking method:

1. Put the dates that have had the pits removed into a blender. Add the cardamom powder, yogurt (or dairy-free yogurt), and almond milk. Blend until smooth.

2. Mix until lumps are eliminated.

3. Combine everything in such a way that it becomes velvety smooth.

4. Place in glass and then finish off with a few date pieces on each one.

5. This cardamom and date smoothie is a wonderful alternative for those looking for a dessert that is both comforting and delicious.

191.   Beet Smoothie

What we need:

- Butter
- 2 tbsp. of pumpkin seeds
- 1 cup beet slices into small pieces
- 2 cups of tea
- 2 tbsp. of linseed
- 2 cups strawberry

Cooking Method:

1. Get all the elements together, and then mix them in the blender.

2. Serve

192. Green Smoothie Bowl

What we need:

- ½ ripe banana
- 1 cup kale
- ¼ cup fresh pineapple chunks
- ½ tsp. fresh ginger
- ½ cup sliced cucumber
- 1 tbsp. of chia seeds
- ½ cup coconut water

Cooking method:

1. Spinach or kale, banana, cucumber slices, fresh ginger, and coconut water should be pureed in a blender until smooth.
2. A bowl is the proper place to pour the smoothie.
3. Chia seeds and fresh pineapple pieces should be sprinkled on top.
4. Take your time to enjoy the reviving tastes as you gently sip.

193. Mango Lassi

What we need:

- Yogurt or dairy-free yogurt
- Crushed pistachios for garnish
- Ripe mangoes, peeled and diced
- Honey (for sweetness)
- Cardamom powder

Cooking method:

1. In a blender, combine ripe mangoes, yogurt, cardamom powder, and honey.
2. Combine until the mixture reaches a velvety consistency.
3. Serve in glasses and top with pistachio crumbles.
4. Dessert doesn't get much more wonderful and refreshing than this Ayurvedic mango lasagna.

30 Days Meal Plan

Day	Breakfast	Lunch	Dinner
1	Baked Egg Cups	Grilled Chicken and Avocado Salad	Sweet Potato and Chickpea Curry
2	Browned Butter Mocha Latte	Deviled Egg with Pickled Jalapenos	Red Lentil and Vegetable Soup
3	Sausage and Egg Sandwich	Banana Porridge	Chickpea and Quinoa Salad
4	Fermented Carrots	Adobo Chicken	Quinoa and Vegetable Stir-Fry
5	Fermented Beetroot	Tofu and Veggie Breakfast Burrito	Cumin-Spiced Carrot Soup
6	Fermented Green Beans	Vegan Curd	Spaghetti Squash with Pesto
7	Fermented Cabbage	Beef Bread	Stuffed Bell Peppers
8	High-Cruciferous Juice	Almond with Coconut	Zucchini Noodles with Pesto
9	Fermented Zucchini	Sweet Potato with Black Bean	Chickpea and Brown Rice Bowl
10	Pineapple and Blueberry Smoothie	Walnut Duck	Cumin-Spiced Carrot Soup
11	Fermented Green Beans	Mixed Berries and Granola	Nut and Fruit Oatmeal
12	Corn Pudding	Banana Porridge	Rice and Vegetable Pilaf
13	Egg and Avocado Salad	Almond with Coconut	Cabbage Porridge with Red Pesto
14	Eggs and Vegetables	Cottage Cheese and Fruit Bowl	Stuffed Bell Peppers
15	Fermented Zucchini	Vegan Curd	Chickpea and Quinoa Salad
16	The Exquisite Greek Yogurt Parfait	Apple Cinnamon Baked Oatmeal	Zucchini Noodles with Pesto
17	Browned Butter Mocha Latte	Vegetable Rice	Tilapia Breaded
18	High-Cruciferous Juice	Coconut Mango Chia Pudding	Cauliflower and Green Bean Stir-Fry
19	Chicken Cashew	Cottage Cheese and Fruit Bowl	Spaghetti Squash with Pesto
20	Quinoa Breakfast Bowl	Adobo Chicken	Greek Salad with Quinoa

21	Fermented Beetroot	Beef Bread	Cabbage Porridge with Red Pesto
22	Chicken Cashew	Tofu and Veggie Breakfast Burrito	Cauliflower and Green Bean Stir-Fry
23	Egg and Avocado Salad	Apple Cinnamon Baked Oatmeal	Red Lentil and Vegetable Soup
24	The Exquisite Greek Yogurt Parfait	Deviled Egg with Pickled Jalapenos	Chickpea and Brown Rice Bowl
25	Fermented Carrots	Walnut Duck	
26	Chickpea and Spinach Curry	Coconut Mango Chia Pudding	Sweet Potato and Chickpea Curry
27	Eggs and Vegetables	Mixed Berries and Granola	Quinoa and Vegetable Stir-Fry
28	Sausage and Egg Sandwich	Vegetable Rice	Greek Salad with Quinoa
29	Corn Pudding	Sweet Potato with Black Bean	Tilapia Breaded
30	Pineapple and Blueberry Smoothie	Grilled Chicken and Avocado Salad	Nut and Fruit Oatmeal

CONCLUSION

In this book, we've explored a variety of nutritious and delicious recipe, each crafted to support a balanced and healthy lifestyle. We design every meal plan and Cooking Method: with care and attention to detail, from hearty breakfasts to satisfying lunches and dinners that fuel your body. By incorporating a wide range of ingredients, including fresh vegetables, lean proteins, and wholesome grains, we've ensured that your diet remains both exciting and nutritionally robust.

The focus on fermented foods and a variety of snacks not only adds diversity to your meals but also promotes gut health and sustained energy levels throughout the day. With recipe that caters to different dietary preferences and requirements, this book aims to make healthy eating accessible and enjoyable for everyone.

This book promotes mindful eating practices and the appreciation of food as a source of both sustenance and pleasure by embracing a balanced approach to nutrition. The recipe books and meal plans offered here are a great tool for reaching your objectives, whether they weight management, general health improvement, or just expanding your culinary horizons.

As you set out on this path to improved health and wellbeing, keep in mind that consistency is essential. Enjoy the process, savor each meal, and celebrate the positive changes that come with a wholesome and balanced diet. Remember, making lasting changes takes time and patience. This book is here to guide you every step of the way, providing you with the tools and inspiration to transform your eating habits and enhance your overall quality of life. Stay committed, be patient with yourself, and enjoy the delicious rewards of a healthier, happier you.

Made in United States
Troutdale, OR
02/04/2025

28672974R00080